"Neuroplasticity? Genetic research? Electromagnetic flow? Never in a million years did I think I could relate to, much less understand, topics like these. Leave me to my normal right-brained tendencies and I'd run as far and fast as I could at the first mention of them. But that was before I met Dr. Caroline Leaf. Some of the most life-transformative lessons I've learned have come from this incredible woman whose brilliance is upstaged only by her integrity and graciousness. Whether sitting in an audience along with twenty thousand other people hanging on to her every word, or just sitting across from her over a couple mugs of hot tea, I've heard her share deeply scientific data in a profoundly practical and simple way that every person can understand. Even me. *Switch On Your Brain* will show you how to turn on the part of your brain, and your life, that has been turned off for far too long. You'll emerge a happier, healthier, and more well-rounded human being."

—Priscilla Shirer, author of *The Resolution for Women*

"Dr. Caroline Leaf masterfully weaves brain science and the Word of God. Not only will *Switch On Your Brain* detox your brain, it will awaken your brilliance—so that you can be all that God created you to be and do all he fashioned you to do. Read it and renew your mind."

—John and Lisa Bevere, authors; cofounders of Messenger International

"I am neither a scientist nor a specialist in this field, but what I do know is that the fruit and influence of Dr. Caroline Leaf's ministry is inspiring people to see—from a scientific perspective—the genius of God's timeless Word and wisdom. Each of us is full of untapped potential when it comes to our ability to think and process our way through life. I pray that Caroline's years of research and passion in this realm of unfolding science will be a blessing to you as you discover what it is to 'switch on your brain.'"

—Bobbie Houston, senior pastor, Hillsong Church

"In *Switch On Your Brain*, my good friend Dr. Caroline Leaf shows us all how the science of thought is catching up with the Word of God. Featuring the 21-Day Brain Detox Plan, Dr. Leaf shares the brain-boosting secrets that she used successfully with thousands of her patients, teaching you how to literally rewire your brain. If you're looking to improve your memory, your focus, your concentration, or your very life, it's time to switch on your brain!"

—Jordan Rubin, NMD, PhD, author of *The Maker's Diet*; founder of Garden of Life and Beyond Organic

"Can you imagine the outcome of a collaborative effort between a brain scientist and a faith-filled believer with a deep biblical foundation? Fortunately, we have the benefit of such resources from someone who possesses an aptitude in both realms. Dr. Caroline's works have provided rare insight into the fascinating inner workings of both the natural and the spiritual. *Switch On Your Brain* underscores that the capacity for abundant living we have through Christ is directly linked to choice. Her teaching provides both exploration and exercises to enable 'the lights to come on,' helping the reader experience a new level of freedom. Her candid and authentic delivery is refreshing and uplifting. I'm grateful for this gift of hope supported by both biblical and scientific proof!"

—Colleen Rouse, pastor of Victory Church Atlanta

"When Dr. Caroline Leaf first appeared on *LIFE Today* in 2007, our viewers were captivated by her research on how humans think. Dr. Leaf connects the dots between science and Scripture—explaining how we can indeed be 'transformed by the renewing of [our] mind.' If you need a change in your thought life or overall attitude, *Switch On Your Brain* will convince you that your brain can be renewed by the power of God's Spirit and biblical truth."

—James Robison, president of LIFE Outreach International;
cohost of *LIFE Today*

"This book is the owner's manual for how our brains work. Caroline Leaf's first appearance on TBN's *Praise the Lord* program with Laurie and myself is one of the 'stuck' memories in my brain. Science in 2013 is actually catching up with the Bible! She has taught us more and more truth over the years now and is in production on an entire TV series that will air on TBN for years!"

—Matt Crouch, broadcaster, filmmaker

"Caroline Leaf has given us a real jewel, translating modern brain science into language accessible to everyone. She engages, educates, and encourages us to use science and biblical truths to improve our thoughts, relationships, and health. This book is a delight, and I highly recommend it to everyone interested in improving their joy and mental health."

—David I. Levy, MD, neurosurgeon; author of *Gray Matter*

"I resolved not to let twelve years of abuse destroy my mind and my life; I resolved not to let injustice flourish on this earth and instead to stand up and do something about it; I decided to make something out of my brokenness; I decided *to choose to change my mind*. Caroline helped me to understand the science behind what had happened in my brain when I made these choices in my life. She explains how our choices work scientifically, but in a practical way that makes something that is really hard to do much easier and more tangible. This book is so helpful that all the girls who go through our A21 program will be learning how to use these principles to help them renew their minds and give them hope so that they can get back into life . . . and change not only their lives but also their world."

—Christine Caine, founder of the A21 Campaign;
director of Equip and Empower Ministries; author of *Undaunted*

"Dr. Leaf has spoken at Gateway on many occasions, and we're so grateful for the impact she's had on our congregation. We've seen firsthand how her unique and groundbreaking message changes lives. She understands that your brain is fearfully and wonderfully made by God. We encourage you to act on the wisdom found in *Switch On Your Brain* and begin the incredible journey of thinking God's way."

—Robert and Debbie Morris, pastors of Gateway Church;
authors of *The Blessed Life*, *The Blessed Marriage*,
and *The Blessed Woman*

"Dr. Caroline Leaf's research allows for tangible understanding of the link between the Bible and the brain and shows us how understanding this develops us both emotionally and spiritually. Her teaching is not only life changing but life *saving* as it makes the renewing of the mind so real. I am so very grateful for the wisdom contained within these pages. Grow as you read."

—Darlene Zschech, singer-songwriter; author of *The Art of Mentoring*

"*Switch On Your Brain* is such a marvelous revelation of how powerful the brain is. I love this! So many times we think, *Well, this is the way I've always been and I can't change.* Not true. No matter how we have thought in the past, we can change our present and future with our thinking. God has told us these things, but Caroline has researched them and proven them scientifically. I believe with all my heart that God wants to soak you in his love and to share the revelation of how to detox your brain from the lies of the enemy and switch it on to the love and truth of God's Word. Thank you, Caroline, for the years you have spent in study, for your commitment to Jesus, for your humility and wisdom, and for being a wonderful friend."

—Marilyn Hickey, president and founder of Marilyn Hickey Ministries

"If our teachers and students could really grasp the power that we each have to think differently, as described by Dr. Caroline Leaf, we could see a true change in education. When each individual, whether adult, teen, or child, begins to take personal responsibility for our own mental, physical, and spiritual health, it will change lives!"

—Angie McDonald, superintendent of Advantage Academy Charter Schools

"In this book Dr. Leaf provides you with the key to detoxifying your brain. She combines her years of expertise in brain research with the Word and wisdom of God to show you that you have the ability to rewire negative thoughts and habits that have led you to live a life of ill health, depression, and defeat. Dr. Leaf includes a 21-Day Brain Detox Plan that will teach you how to get the negativity out of your thinking, allowing you to recalculate your destination from down a negative road to one that leads to a happier, healthier, more productive you. We live or die by the choices we make; but if our brains are toxic from poisonous circumstances, events, and decisions from our past, we cannot make quality choices that will effect positive change until we correct our thinking. I encourage you to take advantage of Dr. Leaf's combination of the Word, wisdom, and science to learn how to 'flip the switch,' enabling you to do, be, and have all that God intended for your life."

—DeeDee Freeman, associate pastor of Spirit of Faith Christian Center

"Our thought life plays a critical role in the outward expression of our being. In *Switch On Your Brain* Caroline Leaf describes how advancements in cognitive neuroscience support biblical principles pertaining to a healthy thought life. She describes how a healthy thought life can have beneficial effects on our overall health and physiology. She provides a practical strategy to align our thought life with biblical truth to facilitate being continually transformed by the renewing of our mind (Romans 12:2). Dr. Leaf challenges us to see ourselves the way God sees us, through the perfect and finished work of Jesus Christ."

—Brian E. Snell, MD, neurosurgeon

"Dr. Leaf demonstrates to us that these breakthroughs in neuroscience are actually ancient, already referenced in the Bible. Neuroscience is actually confirming God's Word. Caroline's gift is her ability to renew our childlike wonder at God's wisdom and creation; we are truly fearfully and wonderfully made (Psalm 139:14). In the second part of the book Dr. Leaf explains how this knowledge can be applied to our lives in a way that even a child can understand. Drawing from her years in clinical practice, she is able to give us practical steps that can truly transform our lives: spirit, soul, and body. I have seen firsthand how these steps have revolutionized people's lives in family, church, and educational settings. Indeed, they have transformed my own life."

—Dr. Peter Amua-Quarshie, MD, MPH, MS, neuroscientist

"When I first met Caroline Leaf in Rwanda years ago, I knew I had met someone with a message that had to be shared with the world. As I leaned in to listen to her heart, her story, her wisdom, and her research, I felt hope rising within me. This is a book of wisdom, knowledge, and truth for everyone. Dr. Leaf's research and insights based on biblical truth give every reader practical keys to live a happy, healthy, and fulfilled life starting today."

—Helen Burns, pastor of Relate Church; author; international speaker; cohost of TV show *Relate with John & Helen Burns*

"Caroline Leaf is such an amazing person, and her book *Switch On Your Brain* is super helpful for everyone because we all need help with our thinking! Dr. Leaf teaches us, in this book, some very essential techniques and insights to help us live a life of peace, health, and happiness. This book will be hugely helpful to you no matter your age or educational background!"

—Sarah Bowling, pastor; cohost with Marilyn Hickey

"I have had the privilege of working with Dr. Leaf when she taught at The King's University in Los Angeles. During the courses she taught, her books were reviewed, critically examined, and thereafter uniformly adopted by course attendees, college and seminary students, and myself. As you will learn, her teachings are on the cutting edge of research in neuroscience. I am enthusiastic about the material in her latest book, as its application can radically change lives and enhance our walk with Jesus. I recommend you read this book, study the material, and apply the teachings. It will begin a great journey."

—C. Fred Cassity, BSE, JD, professor of practical theology, The King's University

"This new book by Caroline Leaf is a practical plan that helps you implement a technique that takes just seven minutes per day to rewire your brain and change your life. I can personally attest to the effectiveness of her methods since I have been healed now for over eight years of several incurable conditions, including autoimmune thyroid disease, acid reflux, fibroid tumors of the uterus, panic attacks, depression, and chronic fatigue syndrome. I was healed through the use of intentional thinking—meditating on the truth to combat the lies about myself and my life that had been programmed into my psyche. I'm not the same person because I have started to think differently. The simple and easy-to-implement concepts in this book can truly change your life. I encourage you to start today!"

—Jennifer Crow, founder of Beautiful Dream Society; author of *Perfect Lies*

"Dr. Leaf has written a book that has the potential to change the life of each of us! Her research and study of the brain has shown that we do have the ability to change our future by changing how we think. In very practical ways she shows us how to do this. This is such an exciting book and I know will be a huge blessing to everyone who reads it!"

—Holly Wagner, pastor of Oasis Church; author of *GodChicks*

# SWITCH ON YOUR BRAIN

## The Key to Peak Happiness, Thinking, and Health

## DR. CAROLINE LEAF

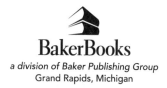

BakerBooks

a division of Baker Publishing Group
Grand Rapids, Michigan

Published by Baker Books
a division of Baker Publishing Group
P.O. Box 6287, Grand Rapids, MI 49516-6287
www.bakerbooks.com

Printed in the United States of America

Library of Congress Cataloging-in-Publication Data
Leaf, Caroline, 1963–
    Switch On Your Brain : The Key to Peak Happiness, Thinking, and Health /
Dr. Caroline Leaf.
        pages cm
    ISBN 978-0-8010-1570-0 (cloth)
    ISBN 978-0-8010-1624-0 (pbk.)
    1. Thought and thinking—Religious aspects—Christianity. 2. Well-being—Religious aspects—Christianity. I. Title.
BV4598.4.L43 2013
248.4—dc23                                                            2013014493

13  14  15  16  17  18  19          7  6  5  4  3  2  1

I see myself as a puzzle builder. And in writing my books, the pieces of the puzzles come together to tell a specific story of hope.

This book is dedicated to:

The ultimate Creator of the puzzles—thank you for honoring me with the task of building a few pieces of the "science of thought" puzzle. I am humbled by this task and will endeavor to bring only you glory through it.

My ever-loving, magnificent love of my life—Mac, my husband. You never seem to tire of listening to me teach on God and the brain with rapt enthusiasm. My sister once said to me that I wouldn't be able to do what I do if it wasn't for you, and this is so true. You are the epitome of loving husbands.

My four outstanding phenomenal children—Jessica, Dominique, Jeffrey, and Alexandria. When I look at you and listen to you, I know I am experiencing God's love and hope and joy. He has blessed me with the epitome of loving children as well.

Our life is what our thoughts make it.

Marcus Aurelius

# Contents

# Contents

# Prologue

W hat would you do if you found a switch that could turn on your brain and enable you to be happier, healthier in your mind and body, more prosperous, and more intelligent?

In this book you will learn how to find and activate that switch. What you think with your mind changes your brain and body, and you are designed with the power to switch on your brain. Your mind is that switch.

You have an extraordinary ability to determine, achieve, and maintain optimal levels of intelligence, mental health, peace, and happiness, as well as the prevention of disease in your body and mind. You can, through conscious effort, gain control of your thoughts and feelings, and in doing so, you can change the programming and chemistry of your brain.

Science is finally catching up with the Bible, showing us the proof that "God has not given us a spirit of fear, but of power and of love and of a sound mind" (2 Tim. 1:7). Breakthrough neuroscientific research is confirming daily what we instinctively knew all along: What you are thinking every moment of every day becomes a physical reality in your brain and body, which affects your optimal mental and physical health. These thoughts collectively form your attitude, which is your state of mind, and it's *your attitude and not your DNA* that determines much of the quality of your life. This state of mind is a real, physical, electromagnetic, quantum, and chemical flow in the brain that switches groups of genes on or off in a positive or negative direction based on your choices and subsequent reactions. Scientifically, this is called *epigenetics*; spiritually, this is the enactment of Deuteronomy 30:19, "I have set before you life and death, blessing and cursing; therefore choose life, that both you and your descendants may live." The brain responds to your mind by sending these neurological signals throughout the body, which means that your thoughts and emotions are transformed into physiological and spiritual effects, and then physiological experiences transform into mental and emotional states. It's a profound and eye-opening thought to realize something seemingly immaterial like a belief can take on a physical existence as a positive or negative change in our cells.

And you are in control of all of this. The choices you make today not only impact your spirit, soul, and body, but can also impact the next four generations.

The great news is that we are *wired for love*, which means all our mental circuitry is wired only for the positive, and we have a natural *optimism bias* wired into us. Our default mode is one of being designed to make good choices. So our bad choices and reactions were wired in by our choices, and therefore can be *wired out*. Our brain is neuroplastic—it can change and regrow. In addition, God has built in the operating principle of neurogenesis—new nerve cells are birthed daily for our mental benefit. This sounds like Lamentations

3:22–23, "The LORD's mercies . . . are new every morning." This book shows you how to *get back control* over your thoughts and renew (as in Rom. 12:2) and rewire your brain in the direction you were originally designed to go.

Based solidly on the latest neuroscientific research on the brain, as well as my clinical experience and research, you will learn how thoughts impact your spirit, soul, and body. You will also learn how to detox your thoughts using my practical, detailed, and easy-to-use 21-Day Brain Detox Plan.

The application is for all walks of life. You won't forgive that person, get rid of that anxiety or depression, follow that essential preventative healthcare, strive to that intellectual level you know you are capable of, follow that dream, eat that organic food, do that diet, be that great parent or husband or wife or friend, get that promotion, or make other changes to create a quality, positive lifestyle—*unless you first choose to get your mind right and switch on your brain.* After all, the ability to think and choose and to use your mind correctly is often the hardest step, but it is the first and most powerful step.

> If you realized how powerful your thoughts are, you would never think a negative thought.
>
> Peace Pilgrim

# Acknowledgments

My inspiration for building these puzzles and the pieces of the puzzle have come from multiple sources:

The inspiration starts and ends with God, always.

The thousands of scientists whose brilliant work I have devoured and spent many thousands of hours pouring over, astounded at the truths God is revealing through them—many of whom I have mentioned in this book and in my references.

The dedicated, driven, and sometimes very broken patients and clients I have had the privilege of working with over the years. I see their mindful determination to succeed pull them up, often to beyond levels they thought they were capable of.

The wise Bible and science teachers I have sat under (and still sit under).

The wonderful Baker Books publishing team—efficiency, excellence, and speed describe their high-standard approach to completing a project.

My very special family, whose love and support have always been a scaffold to me.

My friends: There are so many who have encouraged me and spoken words of wisdom and prophecy over my life, and who contributed to this book in ways they perhaps don't even realize. Mentioning all of you would fill pages, but you know who you are, and I appreciate and love you all. In fact, it was hard to choose who *not* to ask to do endorsements because I wanted all of you in my book.

# Introduction

*Switch On Your Brain with Hope*

> **Main Scripture:** Faith is the substance of things hoped for, the evidence of things not seen. Hebrews 11:1
>
> **Linked Science Concept:** Thoughts are real, physical things that occupy mental real estate. Moment by moment, every day, you are changing the structure of your brain through your thinking. When we hope, it is an activity of the mind that changes the structure of our brain in a positive and normal direction.

It was only a few decades ago that scientists—including those who trained me—considered the brain to be a fixed and hardwired machine. This view saw the damaged brain as incurable. They believed brain damage was hopeless and untreatable, whether the effects were from stroke, cardiovascular event, traumatic brain injury, learning disabilities, traumas, PTSD, OCD, depression, anxiety—even aging. All of these causes and conditions were seen as largely irreversible.

Because this was the presiding view of the brain, I was trained back in the '80s to teach my patients *compensation*, not *restoration* of function. I was trained in the conventional wisdom of the time that said brain normality was an impossibility for those with mental limitations or brain damage of any kind. Being a student of the Bible, however, I was deeply familiar with and constantly comforted by Romans 12:2: "Do not conform to the pattern of this world, but be transformed by the renewing of your mind" (NIV). I knew this famous and fabulous "renewing of the mind" passage was a truth I needed to apply to my patients' care to help them overcome their deficits. So my relentless search of this truth as a scientist began.

I was struck by how my patients, using the therapeutic techniques I was developing from my research, belied the negative picture conventional science presented of the human brain at that time. These results confirmed that the brain, far from being fixed in toxicity, can change even in the most challenging neurological situations.

I was in awe of what each patient displayed in terms of what you *can do when you set your mind to it*. Each new scientific study in this direction confirmed what I knew intuitively to be true: We are not victims of our biology or circumstances. How we react to the events and circumstances of life can have an enormous impact on our mental and even physical health.

As we think, we change the physical nature of our brain. As we consciously direct our thinking, we can wire out toxic patterns of thinking and replace them with healthy thoughts. New thought networks grow. We increase our intelligence and bring healing to our brains, minds, and physical bodies.

It all starts in the realm of the mind, with our ability to think and choose—the most powerful thing in the universe after God, and indeed, fashioned after God.

**Healthy Memory: Adapted Graphic Sketch**

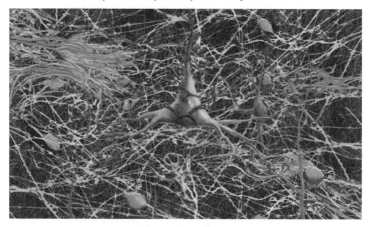

**Toxic Memory: Adapted Graphic Sketch**

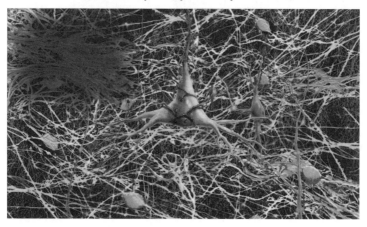

It is with our phenomenal minds that we understand the truths set down in our spirits. It is with our minds that we wire these truths into the brain, which is part of the body. It is with our minds that we choose to develop the spiritual part of who we are and "Therefore put away all filthiness and rampant wickedness and receive with meekness the implanted word, which is able to save your souls" (James 1:21 ESV). It is with our minds that we reject or believe the lies of the Enemy, the Prince of Lies. It is with our minds that we change the physical reality of the brain to reflect our choices. It is with our minds that we decide to follow God's rules and live in peace despite what is going on around us. It is with our minds that we choose to follow the lies of Satan and spiral into mental, physical, and spiritual disarray.

Thought changes the structure of matter. God said, "Let there be light" (Gen. 1:3), and his words produced the physical earth. And science, which, again, is just catching up with the Word of God, is confirming this reality in a tangible and thought-provoking way with eminently clear accounts arising from the burgeoning field of neuroplasticity research.

Neuroplasticity by definition means the brain is malleable and adaptable, changing moment by moment of every day. Scientists are finally beginning to see the brain as having renewable characteristics (as in Rom. 12:2); it is no longer viewed as a machine that is hardwired early in life, unable to adapt, and wearing out with age. With example after fascinating example, exceptional scientists talk about and demonstrate—using brain-imaging techniques and the evidence of behavioral changes—how people can change their brains with their minds. We can see and measure the activity of the mind through the firing of neurons. We can even predict the seeming elusiveness of the main functions of the mind—that of thinking and choosing—through quantum mechanics.

I continue to find myself moving in a world of engrossing truths, and my spirit leaps inside of me. The fact that the brain is plastic and can actually be changed by the mind gives tangible hope to everyone, no matter what the circumstance. I have been privileged to work with and see:

- autistic children cope in academic and social environments
- senior citizens sharpen their memories to the point that in their eighties they change careers and obtain degrees
- young men and women who grew up in abject poverty and a lifestyle of selling and taking drugs do a complete about-face in their lives, go back to school, and become leaders in their communities
- car accident victims who had been written off by neurologists as "vegetables" retrain their brains to the point that they complete their schooling up to a tertiary level and go on to become successful, contributing citizens
- students labeled as learning disabled with years of therapy and no hope left master learning and achieve grades they and their parents only dreamed of
- schools in some of the worst third-world areas in Africa, in which students could not pass to the next level, become schools on the minister of education's "most improved" list
- children with dyslexia learn to read and write and even help their parents study for exams successfully
- suicidal and emotionally traumatized minds set free
- entire schools improve grades across core subjects

And the list goes on.

Science is hovering on a precipice as we recognize the responsibility and impact of our thinking and the resultant choices we make, which have ramifications right down to the ways in which the genes of our bodies express themselves. Deuteronomy 30:19 is becoming a reality in the world we live in today as we begin to see the effects of choice in the brain and body: "I set before you life and death, blessing and cursing; choose life so that you and your descendants may live."

How we think not only affects our own spirit, soul, and body but also people around us. Science and Scripture both show how the results of our decisions pass through the sperm and ova to the next four generations, profoundly affecting their choices and lifestyles. The science of epigenetics (the signals, including our thoughts, that affect the activity of our genes) explains how this plays out. This reminds me of the Scripture, "he punishes the children and their children for the sin of the parents to the third and fourth generation" (Exod. 34:7 NIV).

That the brain is plastic and can be changed moment-by-moment by how we direct our thinking—in other words, the choices we make—is a top idea on the bestseller lists, and it actually is the key to switching on our brains. Add to this the fact that every morning when you wake up, new baby nerve cells have been born while you were sleeping that are there at your disposal to be used in tearing down toxic thoughts and rebuilding healthy thoughts. The birth of these new baby nerve cells is called neurogenesis, which brings to mind, "The Lord's mercies . . . are new every morning" (Lam. 3:23).

What a remarkable and hopeful portrait of the endless adaptivity of the human brain God has given us.

This book is divided into two parts, with the overall goal of showing you how to switch on your brain. Part 1 uncovers the keys to doing so. In part 2 you will see how all these keys work together in my 5-Step Switch On Your Brain Learning Process during my 21-Day Brain Detox Plan. Here I will lead you through a process of switching on your brain to achieve peak happiness, thinking, and health.

Here are some of the key points in this book:

- Your mind is the most powerful thing in the universe after God.
- Free will and choice are real, spiritual, and scientific facts (Deut. 30:19).
- Your mind (soul) has one foot in the door of the spirit and one foot in the door of the body; you can change your brain with your mind and essentially renew your mind (Rom. 12:2).
- You can develop your spirit through choices you make in your mind to be led by the Holy Spirit (Gal. 2:20).
- Your body is not in control of your mind—your mind is in control of your body, and your mind is stronger than your body. Mind certainly is *over* matter.
- You are not a victim of your biology.
- You cannot control the events and circumstances of life, but you can control your reaction to those events and circumstances (Matt. 7:13–14; Gal. 6:7–8).
- When you think, you build thoughts, and these become physical substances in your brain. "As he thinks in his heart, so is he" (Prov. 23:7).
- Good thinking = good choices = healthy thoughts; toxic thinking = toxic choices = toxic thoughts (Deut. 30:19).
- You are designed to stand outside yourself and observe your own thinking *and change it* (Rom. 12:2; 2 Cor. 10:5; Phil. 3:13–14).
- You are designed to recognize and choose the right things to think about (Josh. 24:15; Eccles. 7:29; Isa. 30:2).
- Each morning when you wake up, you have new baby nerve cells born inside your brain to use wisely as you

remove bad thoughts and wire in new ones (Lam. 3:23). This is called neurogenesis.

- You have been designed for deep, intellectual thought (Ps. 139:14).
- You are wired for love, and fear is a learned and not a natural response (2 Tim. 1:7).
- You have the mind of Christ (1 Cor. 2:16).
- You are made in God's image (Gen. 1:27).

All this knowledge will help you realize these truths:

- Happiness comes from within and success follows—not the other way around.
- You can learn how to learn and deepen your intellect.
- You can overcome those learning issues.
- You can get the chaos in your mind under control.
- You don't have to walk around in guilt and condemnation.
- If you wired those toxic thoughts in, you can wire them out.
- You don't have to get stuck in bad habits; you can change them.
- You can overcome feelings of rejection and hurt.
- Forgiveness is not the battle you think it is.
- You don't have to worry about things that are out of your control.
- You are not a victim of the things you shouldn't be doing.
- You don't have to fear that if a condition runs in your family that you are going to get it (for example, Alzheimer's, Parkinson's, or depression).

- You can balance your over-thinking and over-analyzing mind.

- You can overcome and control depression and anxiety—some scientists are showing you can even control and overcome schizophrenia and OCD.

- You don't have to keep digging into the past to get free from it.

- You can be happy and filled with peace regardless of your circumstances.

If you have nodded your head at even one of these, it is time for you to be set free in your mind to pursue all God has for you. Read on. It is time for you to Switch On Your Brain and find the keys to peak happiness, thinking, and health.

In part 1, I explain through science and Scripture how the concepts described above come together.

In part 2, you will find my 21-Day Brain Detox Plan, which incorporates my scientifically proven 5-Step Switch On Your Brain technique based on my research, my years in clinical practice, and doing seminars and conferences around the world. This section is practical and filled with key, proven strategies that will help you develop a lifestyle of renewing your mind and aligning it with God's will so your divine sense of purpose can be released (Eccles. 3:11).

You are truly designed for peak happiness, thinking, and health.

## Introduction Summary

1. It was only a few decades ago that scientists considered the brain to be a fixed and hardwired machine. This

view saw the damaged brain as incurable and the focus was *compensation*, not restoration of function.

2. We can change the physical nature of our brain through our thinking and choosing.

3. As we consciously direct our thinking, we can wire out toxic patterns of thinking and replace them with healthy thoughts. New thought networks grow. We increase our intelligence and bring healing to our minds and physical bodies.

4. It *all* starts in the realm of the mind, with our ability to think and choose—the most powerful thing in the universe after God.

5. Neuroplasticity by definition means the brain is malleable and adaptable, changing moment by moment of every day.

6. Scientists are finally beginning to see the brain as having renewable characteristics (as in Rom. 12:2).

7. Science is hovering on a precipice as we recognize the responsibility and impact of our thinking and the resultant choices we make, which have ramifications right down to the ways in which the genes of our bodies express themselves.

8. Neurogenesis is the birth of new baby nerve cells.

## PART 1

# How to Switch On Your Brain

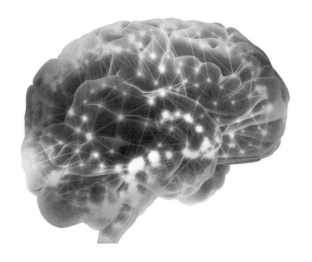

# 1

# Mind Controls Matter

Main Scripture: God has not given us a spirit of fear, but of power and of love and of a sound mind. 2 Timothy 1:7

Linked Science Concept: Science shows we are wired for love with a natural optimism bias. This means exactly what the Scripture says above.

The debate in science is between the mind being what the brain does versus the brain doing the bidding of the mind. The position you adopt will impact how you view free will and choice.

## The Mind Is What the Brain Does

The first argument proposes that thoughts come from your brain as though your brain is generating all aspects of your mental experience. People who hold this view are called the *materialists*. They believe that it is the chemicals and neurons that create the mind and that the relationships between your thoughts and what you do can just be ignored.

So essentially, their perspective is that the brain creates what you are doing and what you are thinking. The mind is what the brain does, they believe, and the ramifications are significant. Take, for example, the treatment of depression. In this reductionist view depression is a chemical imbalance problem of a machinelike brain; therefore, the treatment is to add in the missing chemicals.

This view is biblically and scientifically incorrect.

## The Brain Does the Bidding of the Mind

Let's look at this from the other angle of the argument: The brain is what the mind does.

You are a thinking being. You think all day long, and at night as you sleep, you sort out your thinking. As you think, you choose, and as you choose, you cause genetic expression to happen in your brain. This means you make proteins, and these proteins form your thoughts. Thoughts are real, physical things that occupy mental real estate.

Eric R. Kandel, a Nobel Prize–winning neuropsychiatrist for his work on memory, shows how our thoughts, even our imaginations, get "under the skin" of our DNA and can turn certain genes on and certain genes off, changing the structure of the neurons in the brain.[1] So as we think and imagine, we change the structure and function of our brains. Even Freud speculated back in the 1800s that thought leads to changes in the brain.[2] In recent years, leading neuroscientists like Marion Diamond, Norman Doidge, Joe Dispenza, Jeffrey Schwartz, Henry Markram, Bruce Lipton, and Allan Jones, to name just a few, have shown how our thoughts have remarkable power to change the brain.[3] Our brain is changing moment by moment as we are thinking. By our thinking and choosing, we are redesigning the landscape of our brain.

Our mind is designed to control the body, of which the brain is a part, not the other way around. Matter does not control us; we control matter through our thinking and choosing. We cannot control the events and circumstances of life but we can control our reactions. In fact, we can control our reactions to anything, and in doing so, we change our brains. It's not easy; it is hard work, but it can be done through our thoughts and choices. This is what I focus on in the second half of the book with my 21-Day Brain Detox Plan.

For now, rest in the assurance that what God has empowered you to do with your mind is more powerful and effective than any medication, any threat, any sickness, or any neurological challenge. The Scripture is clear on this: You do not have a spirit of fear but of love, power, and a sound mind (2 Tim. 1:7). We are not bound by the physical; we control the physical. You just have to look at the many inspirational survival stories of those who have overcome impossible odds throughout history and in the current day to know this is truth.

## Choices Are Real

You are free to make choices about how you focus your attention, and this affects how the chemicals and proteins and wiring of your brain change and function. Scientists are proving that the relationship between what you think and how you understand yourself—your beliefs, dreams, hopes, and thoughts—has a huge impact on how your brain works.

Research shows that 75 to 98 percent of mental, physical, and behavioral illness comes from one's thought life.[4]

This staggering and eye-opening statistic means only 2 to 25 percent of mental and physical illnesses come from the environment and genes.

## Thinking Activates Genes

Every day scientists are discovering the precise pathways by which changes in human consciousness produce changes in our brain and bodies. Our consciousness—this phenomenal gift from God to be able to think—activates our genes and changes our brain. Science shows that our thoughts, with their embedded feelings, turn sets of genes on and off in complex relationships. We take facts, experiences, and the events of life, and assign meaning to them with our thinking.

We may have a fixed set of genes in our chromosomes, but which of those genes are active and *how* they are active has a great deal to do with how we think and process our experiences. Our thoughts produce words and behaviors, which in turn stimulate more thinking and choices that build more thoughts in an endless cycle.

## Our Brains Are Shaped by Our Reactions

We are constantly reacting to circumstances and events, and as this cycle goes on, our brains become shaped by the process in either a positive, good-quality-of-life direction or a negative, toxic, poor-quality-of-life direction. So it is the quality of our thinking and choices (consciousness) and our reactions that determine our "brain architecture"—the shape or design of the brain and *resultant* quality of the health of our minds and bodies.

Science and Scripture both show that we are wired for love and optimism[5] and so when we react by thinking negatively and making negative choices, the quality of our thinking suffers, which means the quality of our brain architecture suffers. It is comforting—and challenging—to know that negative thinking is not the norm.

## Thinking Changes Our DNA

Taking this to a deeper level, research shows that *DNA actually changes shape according to our thoughts.* As you think those negative thoughts about the future—the week ahead, what a person might say or do, even in the absence of the concrete stimulus—that toxic thinking will change your brain wiring in a negative direction and throw your mind and body into stress.[6]

According to Dr. Herbert Benson, MD, president of Harvard Medical School's Mind-Body Institute, negative thinking leads to stress, which affects our body's natural healing capacities.[7]

Toxic thinking wears down the brain.

The Institute of HeartMath, an internationally recognized, nonprofit research organization that helps people reduce stress, discusses an experiment titled "Local and Nonlocal Effects of Coherent Heart Frequencies on Conformational Changes of DNA." This study showed that thinking and feeling anger, fear, and frustration caused DNA to change shape according to thoughts and feelings. The DNA responded by tightening up and becoming shorter, switching off many DNA codes, which reduced quality expression. So we feel shut down by negative emotions, and our body feels this too. But here's the great part: the negative shutdown or poor quality of the DNA codes was *reversed* by feelings of love, joy, appreciation, and gratitude! The researchers also found that HIV positive patients who had positive thoughts and feelings had 300,000 times more resistance to the disease than those without positive feelings.[8] So the takeaway here is that when we operate in our normal love design—which is being made in God's image (Gen. 1:26)—we are able to change the shape of our DNA for the better.

So when we make a poor-quality decision—when we choose to engage toxic thoughts (for example, unforgiveness, bitterness, irritation, or feelings of not coping)—we change the DNA and subsequent genetic expression, which then changes the shape of our brain wiring in a negative direction. This immediately puts the brain into protection mode, and the brain translates these poor-quality, toxic thoughts as negative stress. This stress then manifests in our bodies. But the most exciting part of this study was the hope it demonstrated because the positive attitude, the good choice, rewired everything back to the original healthy positive state. These scientists basically proved we can renew our minds.

## Stress

Stress stage one is normal. This is our alert state that keeps us focused and conscious and is the state we are in when we are thinking in alignment with God. Stress stage two and stage three, however, are our mind and body's response to toxic thinking—normal stress gone wrong. Even a little bit of these negative levels of stress from a little bit of toxic thinking has far-reaching consequences for mental and physical health.

The dictionary defines *stress* as "a condition typically characterized by symptoms of mental and physical tension or strain, as depression or hypertension, that can result from a *reaction* to a situation in which a person feels threatened, pressured, etc."[9] Synonyms for stress include anxiety, nervousness, fearfulness, apprehensiveness, impatience, fear, tenseness, and restlessness.

*Reaction* is the key word here. *You cannot control the events or circumstances of your life, but you can control your reactions.* And controlling those reactions is the difference between healthy minds and bodies and sick minds and bodies. Here are just a few statistics confirming that 75 to 98 percent of mental and physical illness comes from one's thought life:

- A study by the American Medical Association found that stress is a factor in 75 percent of all illnesses and diseases that people suffer from today.[10]

- The association between stress and disease is a colossal 85 percent.[11]

- The International Agency for Research on Cancer and the World Health Organization[12] have concluded that 80 percent of cancers are due to lifestyle and not genetics, and this is a conservative number.

- According to Dr. Bruce Lipton, a scientist who has made great strides in understanding the effect of our thinking on our brain,[13] gene disorders like Huntington's chorea, beta thalassemia, and cystic fibrosis, to name a few, affect less than 2 percent of the population. This means the vast majority of the world's population comes into this world with genes that should enable them to live happy and healthy lives. Lipton says a staggering 98 percent of diseases are related to lifestyle choices—in other words, our thinking.

- According to Dr. H. F. Nijhout,[14] genes control biology and not the other way around.

- According to W. C. Willett,[15] only 5 percent of cancer and cardiovascular patients can attribute their disease to hereditary factors.

- The American Institute of Health estimates that 75–90 percent of all visits to primary care physicians are for stress-related problems.[16] Some of the latest negative stress statistics causing illness as a result of toxic thinking are eye-opening.

The main point of this chapter is that mind controls matter. If we get this right, we have enormous potential to reach peak health. If we get it wrong, we will be our own worst enemies.

## Chapter 1 Summary

1. The debate in science is between the mind being what the brain does versus the brain doing the bidding of the mind.
2. The correct view is that the mind is designed to control the body, of which the brain is a part, not the other way around.
3. Our brain does not control us; we control our brain through our thinking and choosing.
4. We can control our reactions to anything.
5. Choices are real. You are free to make choices about how you focus your attention, and this affects how the chemicals, proteins, and wiring of your brain change and function.
6. Research shows that *DNA actually changes shape in response to our thoughts.*
7. Stress stage one is normal. Stress stage two and stage three, on the other hand, are our mind and body's response to toxic thinking—basically normal stress gone wrong.
8. *Reaction* is the key word here. You cannot control the events or circumstances of your life, but you can control your reactions.

# 2

# Choice and Your Multiple-Perspective Advantage

**Main Scripture:** Let the peace (soul harmony which comes) from Christ rule (act as umpire continually) in your hearts [deciding and settling with finality all questions that arise in your minds, in that peaceful state] to which as [members of Christ's] one body you were also called [to live]. And be thankful (appreciative), [giving praise to God always]. Colossians 3:15 AMP

**Linked Science Concept:** Choice is real, and free will exists. You are able to stand outside of yourself, observe your own thinking, consult with God, and change the negative, toxic thought or grow the healthy, positive thought. When you do this, your brain responds with a positive neurochemical rush and structural changes that will improve your intellect, health, and peace. You will experience soul harmony.

These are obvious statements; however, many of us walk through life as though we are victims of the events and circumstances of life and biology and whatever or whomever else we can think of to blame. As a therapist for nearly twenty-two years and having reached millions of people through my seminars, books, and media appearances, the statements I make more than any others are these: "You are not a victim. You can control your reactions. You do have a choice."

## Free Will Is Not an Illusion

All of us, including God-fearing Christians, fall prey to media proclamations by neuroscientists and researchers who make the news with such leading questions as, "Is free will an illusion?" The problem, however, is that this point of view cannot be reconciled with what we know about the human brain and what Scripture says about us as humans. In a *New York Times* article, a legal analyst even asked, "Because our brains cause all behavior, could all behavior be potentially excused?"[1]

This is dangerous thinking. They are basically saying that we are not responsible for our actions, which provides an excuse to do whatever we want to do with no consequences.

We must always remember that scientists are not God—though they sometimes act like they are. I am a scientist, and if I can't back up a scientific "fact" with Scripture, I question its validity.

Philosophers and scientists have long debated whether we have free will. Some argue free will is a quaint, old-fashioned idea. Of course, the mere fact that people debate this issue means they are using their free will to formulate their opinions and choose their answers. So they quite literally destroy their own argument.

A typical neuroscientist might argue that free decisions are determined ahead of time by brain activity. This argument says the brain is like a machine that has all these programs running, over which we have no control. This machine produces the mind, and we go through life helplessly at the will and mercy of these programs. Then neuroscientists use brain imaging and fancy terminology to argue that free will is just an illusion.

## We Can Choose to Think the Way God Wants Us to Think

As a communication pathologist specializing in the field of cognitive neuroscience, my research is concerned mainly with how humans think and the impact of this thinking on what they say and do, and I have come to a very different conclusion from those who think free will is just an illusion. I'm convinced beyond all doubt that our God-given ability to think and choose means that our free will influences our thinking, which produces our state of mind. This is so important to human behavior and potential that I have dedicated my life to understanding the process of thought and how we can choose to think the way God wants us to think. Far from explaining away free will, the neuroscientific evidence actually explains how free will works.

Molecular biologist Francis Crick, who won a Nobel Prize in 1962 with James Watson for their discovery of DNA in 1953, said free will is "a simple-minded bit of confabulation" and dismissed it as "an exercise in self-delusion."[2] In making this statement, Crick overlooked something important: *He chose with his free will* to formulate that thought and express it.

## Proving Free Will

Brain activity can be identified in the prefrontal cortex (just above the eyebrows) and parietal cortex (top side of your

41

head) seven to ten seconds before an actual decision is verbal-
ized or enacted. Many scientists use this fact to argue that
the decision was already encoded.[3] I see it differently, and I
am in good company with scientists like Jeffrey Schwartz,
Norman Doidge, and others.

My argument is that this brain activity is the processing
activity we do unconsciously, on the very real and active
nonconscious level (see chap. 8), which is flavored by the
thoughts—memories—we have implanted into our nonconscious minds over time. In this phase we choose to add our
own unique perception, based on these implanted thoughts
that form our point of view, on our way to verbalization or
action we perform. So in simple terms, what we say and do
is based on what we have already built into our minds. We
evaluate this information and make our choices based on this
information, then we choose to build a new thought, and this
is what drives what we say or do.

This brain activity, seen in brain imaging, is not the result
of machine-like activity; it is simply the build-up to the moment of consciousness. It is the activity of a network of neural
circuits that begin to prepare for an upcoming decision long
before it enters our awareness. It is the intellectualizing that is
happening in the nonconscious mind. In other words, "As he
thinks in his heart, so is he" (Prov. 23:7). We are not driven by
forces beyond our conscious control. We are accountable for
every thought and decision we make.[4] We are highly intelligent
beings with free will, and we are responsible for our choices.

Some forward-thinking researchers have found that when
people doubt free will, they become more dishonest. It is
almost as though denying free will provides the ultimate excuse to behave however people want without accountability
for their actions.[5]

Other researchers found that believing in free will guides people's choices toward being more moral and better performers. They go so far as to say that the more researchers investigate free will, the more reasons there are to believe in it, and that to an extent those who believe otherwise delude themselves.

Ecclesiastes 7:29 (NLT) says it like this: "God created people to be virtuous, but they have each turned to follow their own downward path." A standard definition of free will is a "set of capacities for imagining future courses of action, deliberating about one's reason for choosing them, planning one's actions in light of this deliberation and controlling actions in the face of competing desires."[6] This, I believe, is how we choose to follow either God's path or Satan's path.

Science is proving free will right down to the genetic level. Let's take a look at some of the evidence.

## Choice Has Mental *Real Estate*

Choice has mental "real estate" around the front of the brain. It includes many circuits that start at the basal forebrain (between your eyebrows) and extend back across the frontal lobe, which is capable of an impressive array of functions and is connected to all other parts of the brain. It is also where connections from all the other parts of the brain converge. Specific circuits go to structures like the insula, corpus callosum, anterior and posterior central gyrus, basal ganglia, precuneus, and subgenuel region of the brain.[7] This arrangement enables the frontal lobe to integrate and manage activities in the other parts of the brain.

## We Can Observe Our Own Thoughts

One of the most exciting features of frontal lobes is how they enable us in a sense to stand outside ourselves and observe

# Inside the Brain

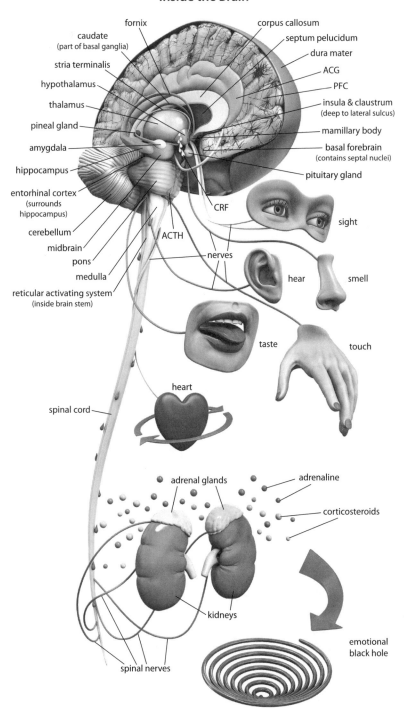

fornix
caudate (part of basal ganglia)
stria terminalis
hypothalamus
thalamus
pineal gland
amygdala
hippocampus
entorhinal cortex (surrounds hippocampus)
cerebellum
midbrain
pons
medulla
reticular activating system (inside brain stem)

corpus callosum
septum pelucidum
dura mater
ACG
PFC
insula & claustrum (deep to lateral sulcus)
mamillary body
basal forebrain (contains septal nuclei)
pituitary gland

CRF
ACTH
nerves
sight
hear
smell
taste
touch
heart
spinal cord

adrenal glands
adrenaline
corticosteroids
kidneys
spinal nerves

emotional black hole

our own thinking. We can observe our thoughts and actions and make decisions about them. Suddenly, biblical principles such as "bringing all thoughts into captivity," "renewing your mind," "casting all your cares," and "being anxious for nothing" become less difficult when we realize God has given us the equipment to do these things.

When we choose life (Deut. 30:19), the diamond increases its shine; when we choose anything other than life, the diamond loses its shine. This is a simple analogy of what happens in the brain. The wrong choices cause brain damage. The right choices enhance brain function.

## Our MPA

We have what I like to call "multiple-perspective advantage"—MPA for short. Our unique, multifaceted nature, made in God's image, allows us to see things from many different angles—like different perspectives. We have the unique opportunity to assess our thoughts and their impact and choose to connect to the vine that is Christ (John 15:1–5)—to restore growth and prune off the branches of toxic thinking.

We are directly responsible for what we choose to think about and dwell on, and we make these decisions in the privacy of our own thinking. As you think, it is important to make a distinction between who you truly are—the real, multifaceted, unique you—and the person you have become through toxic choices. Fortunately, you can see both and choose to reconnect with the vine (John 15) and renew your mind (Rom. 12:2). Your brain will follow the instructions and choices of your mind and change its landscape accordingly. Part 2 of this book will help you do just that.

## The Seven Different Types of Thinking

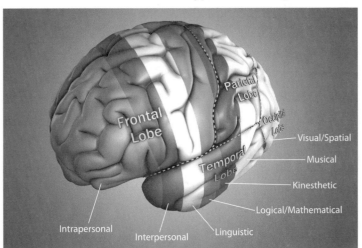

## You Are a Thinking Being

Let's go deeper into the brain to see how influential and real your free will and choices are. You are a thinking being; you think all day long, and you are even thinking while you sleep. Daytime thinking is a building process, whereas nighttime thinking is a sorting process. As you think, you are making your way to a decision of some kind, whether it's as simple as what to eat or as complex as choosing one of several different courses of action you face.

### All Thinking Activity Is Real

All this thinking activity is real, and it can be seen on various types of brain imaging. When we think, marvelous, wondrously complex, and creative things take place. Even if you don't fully understand what I am saying in the next few paragraphs, be in awe of how intricately God has made us.

Just the mind activity from your reading of the next few lines generates electromagnetic, electrochemical, and quantum action in your neurons. It causes

- magnetic fields that can be measured;
- electrical impulses that can be tracked;
- chemical effects that can be seen and measured;
- photons to be activated that can be captured on computer screens;
- energy activity that can be explained using quantum physics; and
- vibrations in the membranes of the neurons that can be picked up by instrumentation.

This combined activity sets up an intricate and organized sequence of actions of neurotransmitters, proteins, and energy that forms a signal. Your thinking has just created a powerful signal that is going to change the landscape of your brain.

### You Create Signals

This signal you have just created passes through the membrane of the cell, travels to the cell's nucleus, and enters the chromosome, activating a strand of DNA. The DNA is zipped up, almost as though it is in a cocoon, until activated or unzipped by the signal. When the DNA is zipped up, it is in a dormant or inert state. This cocoon also protects the DNA from the rest of the intracellular environment while in this inert state.

So, the zipped up DNA has to be opened so that the appropriate genetic code needed to build the protein can be read. As it is opened and the code is read, RNA (a type of protein that almost acts like a photocopier) makes a *photocopy* of the code, which serves as a guide or architectural plan to build the proteins within the *machinery* inside the cell. This is called "genetic expression." And these proteins you have caused to be built hold the information you have just read as a thought or a memory. You have created substance.

Molecules are assembled into protein by the genetic instructions in our DNA. These instructions dictate the anatomy and physiology of our bodies, and we control up to 90 percent of this process through our thinking.

While scientists have brilliantly mapped the whole sequence of gene expression and protein assembly, they have given very little attention to the signals that get the whole thing going in the first place.[8]

## The Signal That Unzips DNA

Let's take a closer look at these signals.

1. The initiating signals that get the ball rolling come from outside the DNA and are therefore called *epigenetic phenomena*, which means signals that control the genes, so they are *epi*—or over and above—the genes.[9]
2. When there is interference with this signal (for example, thinking a toxic thought or eating unhealthy food), genetic expression does not happen correctly and then proteins do not form like they should. So, on a very simplified level, if you have a toxic thought, the resulting proteins look different and act differently than if you had a healthy thought.

3. These signals are electromagnetic and chemical because there is an electromagnetic and chemical component to every biological process.

4. These signals can come from the environment inside the body—the emotional, biochemical, mental, energy, and spiritual, including from the thought networks inside your brain. Or they can come from the environment outside the body—the food, toxins, social network, and nurturing you receive.[10]

Researchers estimate that about 90 percent of genes in the DNA are working with these signals from these outer and inner environments.[11]

## The Switch Gene

One of the many amazing things Kandel discovered was that we have a *switch gene* called the "creb gene," which we *choose* to switch on with our thoughts. So our thoughts are the signal I am talking about in the paragraph above. I wish I could delve further into this fascinating topic, but it is a highly complex process and beyond the purpose of this book, which is not meant to be a scientific tome. However, it is still worth a brief and simple mention because it highlights how God built choice into every sophisticated detail of our being and, once again, gives us the opportunity to admire him.

Here is a simple explanation of this switch gene: As information in the form of electromagnetic and chemical signals moves toward the front part of the brain, it becomes amplified and highly active. This stimulates the release of specialized proteins inside the cell, turning on the creb gene, which acts like a light switch that we choose to switch on or off by our thoughts. This switch creb gene then activates genetic expression (the making of proteins), and we *grow* protein branches that hold our memories, which can also be called our thoughts.[12] So when we choose to switch on the creb gene because of the thoughts we allow to permeate our brain, protein synthesis happens and a new branch grows and makes a connection at a synapse to other branches.

## What Does All This Science Mean to You?

All this scientific and biological information is to say two things:

1. Scientific investigation is a way of admiring God. We admire God's grace and greatness when we get a glimpse at how he has made us and constructed the world we live in. This can give us a sense of peace that he is in control.

2. Scientists are discovering precise pathways by which changes in human thinking operate as signals that activate genetic expression, which then produce changes in our brains and bodies. Our genetic makeup fluctuates by the minute based on what we are thinking and choosing. Clearly, then, following the advice of Philippians 4:8 will have a profound healing and regenerative impact on our bodies and minds by affecting our genetic expression: "Finally, brothers and sisters, whatever is true, whatever is noble, whatever is right, whatever is pure, whatever is lovely, whatever is admirable—if anything is excellent or praiseworthy—think about such things" (NIV). Make this truth your life choice.

## What Does the Future of Medicine Potentially Hold?

Eric Kandel, the Nobel Prize winner for his research on memory, says the following concerning treating patients in the future: "Social influences will be biologically incorporated into the altered expression of specific genes in specific nerve cells of specific areas of the brain."[13] So a time is coming when medical practitioners will include admonitions like Philippians 4:8 and Romans 12:2 on their prescription pads. Part 2 of this book is designed to help you apply God's prescription.

## From the Gene Myth to the Truth

We have been living under a myth called the *gene myth*, which locates the ultimate power over health and mental well-being in the untouchable realm of genes, relegating them to the level of gods. This myth has bound the mental and physical health as well as the peace and happiness of too many people for too long. Almost daily another headline pops up with the highly fashionable concept of a gene for this or a gene for that. You are an alcoholic or depressed or battle with learning disabilities because you have the gene for alcoholism or depression or learning disabilities or whatever. Genes may create an environment within us in which a problem may grow, a predisposition, but they do not produce the problem; we produce it through our choices. Our choices act as the signals that unzip the DNA, which I spoke about earlier in this chapter.

Genes have been made out to be responsible for feelings, spirituality, beliefs—even things like the enjoyment of music—all human behavior, to the extent of determining human affairs, human relationships, and social problems.[14] In fact, genetic predisposition has become entrenched in popular

51

culture to the extent that phrases like "she has good genes" and "he was born that way" are commonplace.

This thinking removes choice and accountability from the equation and is scientifically and spiritually inaccurate. You control your genes; your genes do not control you. Genes may determine physical characteristics but not psychological phenomena. On the contrary, our genes are constantly being remodeled in response to life experiences.[15]

Outstanding research has recently been done by Dr. Gail Ironson, a leading mind-body medicine researcher and professor of psychology and psychiatry at the University of Miami.[16] She found that the most significant factor that made a difference in healing for those with HIV was their choice to believe in a benevolent and loving God, especially if they also chose to have a personal relationship with a benevolent and loving God. Her study ran over four years and her determination of healing was based on the decrease of their viral load, the amount of the AIDS virus in a sample of blood, and the increased concentration of "helper T-cells"—the higher the concentration, the more the body is able to fight disease. She found that those who did not believe God loved them lost helper T-cells three times faster. Their viral load also increased three times faster, and their stress levels were higher, with damaging amounts of cortisol flowing. Dr. Ironson summarizes her research by saying, "If you believe God loves you, it's an enormously protective factor, even more protective than scoring low for depression or high for optimism. A view of a benevolent God is protective, but scoring high on the *personalized* statement 'God loves *me*' is even stronger."[17]

As you can imagine, the implications of this research are enormous, from how we present ourselves to others to how we help others and ourselves manage illness. Our choices have an impact. Our choices become *physiology*, and what we believe as well as what we believe about ourselves alters the facts.

We are not victims of our biology. We are co-creators of our destiny alongside God. God leads, but we have to choose to let God lead. We have been designed to create thoughts, and from these we live out our lives (Prov. 23:7).

Hebrews 11:1 says, "Faith is the substance of things hoped for, the evidence of things not seen." Whatever you believe in and hope for becomes substance on a physical level, and you act upon this. This process can move in either direction—negative or positive.

In the next chapter we look more in depth at the impact of our choices and how to eliminate toxic choices.

## Chapter 2 Summary

1. You are not a victim. You can control your reactions. You do have a choice.
2. Free will is not an illusion. Thinking it is an illusion is dangerous thinking, and it basically says that we are not responsible for our actions, thus providing an excuse to do whatever we want to do, with no consequences.
3. Our free will influences our thinking, which produces our state of mind. This is so important to human behavior and potential that I have dedicated my life to understanding the process of thought and how we can choose to think the way God wants us to think. Far from explaining away free will, the neuroscientific evidence actually explains how free will works.
4. What we say and do is based on what we have already built into our minds. We evaluate this information and

make our choices based on this information. Then we choose to build a new thought, and this is what drives what we say and do.

5. Choice has mental *real estate* around the front of the brain. Certain areas light up when we think and choose.

6. One of the most exciting features of frontal lobes is how they enable us in a sense to stand outside ourselves and observe our own thinking.

7. We have what I like to call "multiple-perspective advantage"—MPA for short. Our unique, multifaceted nature, made in God's image, allows us to see things from many different angles or perspectives.

8. All this thinking activity is real, and it can be seen on various types of brain imaging.

9. This *thinking* creates signals that unzip the DNA, which then expresses genes making proteins.

10. We have a switch gene called the "creb gene" that we choose to switch on with our thoughts.

11. Our genetic makeup fluctuates by the minute based on what we are thinking and choosing.

12. A time is coming when medical practitioners will include admonitions like Philippians 4:8 and Romans 12:2 on their prescription pads. Part 2 of this book is designed to help you apply God's prescription.

13. From the gene myth to the truth: We are not victims of our biology; we control our biology.

# 3

# Your Choices
# Change Your Brain

**Main Scripture:** Do not conform to the pattern of this world, but be transformed by the renewing of your mind. Then you will be able to test and approve what God's will is—his good, pleasing and perfect will. Romans 12:2 NIV

**Linked Science Concept:** Through our thoughts we can be our own micro surgeons as we make choices that will change the circuits in our brains. We are designed to do our own brain surgery and rewire our brains by thinking and by choosing to renew our minds.

Our choices—the natural consequences of our thoughts and imagination—get "under the skin" of our DNA and can turn certain genes on and off, changing the structure of the neurons in our brains. So our thoughts, imagination, and choices can change the structure and function of our brains on every level: molecular, genetic, epigenetic, cellular, structural, neurochemical, electromagnetic, and even subatomic. Through our thoughts, we can be our own brain surgeons as we make choices that change the circuits in our brains. We are designed to do our own brain surgery.

This scientific power of our mind to change the brain is called *epigenetics* and spiritually it is as a man thinks, so is he (Prov. 23:7). The way the brain changes as a result of mental activity is scientifically called *neuroplasticity*. And spiritually, it is the renewing of the mind (Rom. 12:2).

In chapter 2, I introduced you to the science of epigenetics, which is tangible, scientific proof of how important our choices are; they bring life or death, blessing or cursing; and they reach beyond us to influence the next generations (Deut. 30:19). This is because choices become signals that change our brain and body, so these changes are not dictated by our genes. Our thinking and subsequent choices become the signal switches for our genes. What's incredible is that genes are dormant until switched on by a signal; they have potential, but they have to be activated to release that potential. They have to be unzipped. (See chap. 2.)

## Epigenetics Is an Ancient Science and Spiritual Truth

Epigenetics is referred to as a new science, but actually it is an ancient science that we find throughout the Bible. At its most basic level, epigenetics is the fact that your thoughts and choices impact your physical brain and body, your mental health, and your spiritual development (Deut. 30:19; Ps. 34:11–16; Prov. 3:7–8). And these choices will impact not only your *own* spirit, soul, and body but also the people with whom you have relationships. In fact, it goes even deeper; your choices might impact the generations that follow: "For the sin of the parents to the third and fourth generation" (Exod. 34:7 NIV; see also Exod. 20:1–6; Num. 14:8; Deut. 5:9).

The decisions you make today become part of the thought networks in your brain. The two copies of the chromosome that you carry in each of your cells contain the entire set of genetic material necessary to make you. An interesting point: A cell in your brain and a cell in your kidney contain the exact same DNA. And while in utero (in the womb), the nascent (emerging, developing) cells differentiate into either a brain cell or a kidney cell *only* when crucial epigenetic processes turn the right genes on or off. So God has designed perfectly timed epigenetic signals to switch on in the womb as the baby is developing. "Before I formed you in the womb I knew you" (Jer. 1:5).

## Our Thoughts Can Impact the Next Four Generations

Science has demonstrated how the thought networks pass through the sperm and the ova via DNA to the next four generations.

One of the first studies showing that an epigenetic signal can affect genetic expression was done with mice that had the agouti gene, which caused them to be fat, have a yellow coat, and have an increased incidence of cancer and diabetes. When the agouti gene occurs in humans, it is related to obesity and type 2 diabetes. In the experiment, just before conception, the agouti mother mice were fed a nutritional chemical called a methyl group in the form of a B vitamin. This acts as a methyl donor, which suppresses the gene expression, with the result that the offspring of this group did not get fat or yellow. So an external signal—the nutritional methyl—changed the generational pattern.[1]

This landmark study fostered a host of studies—including some done on humans—that showed that not only does food change generational patterns, but so does thinking.[2] In 2003 the Human Epigenome project was launched, which showed that epigenetics had moved from being a sideshow back in the 1970s to what is now a main show in the biological arena, putting genetics in a more proportional place.[3]

## Scientific Mysteries

Epigenetics explains certain scientific mysteries that traditional genetics never could—for example, why one member of a pair of identical twins develops asthma but the other does not. They have the same genome, so they should respond the same way, but their individual perception of the world (what I term the "I-factor") as well as their ability to choose means they think and react differently, which alters their genetic expression. Although their genes are the same, their *patterns of expression can be tweaked* through the signal. And this signal is mainly affected by our reaction to the events and circumstances of life. This is profound and the implications are enormous: the way we react—our thinking and choosing—becomes the signal that activates or deactivates the generational issues in our lives.

## The Good, the Bad, and the Ugly

Taken collectively, the studies on epigenetics show us that the good, the bad, and the ugly do come down through the generations, but your mind is the signal—the epigenetic factor—that switches these genes on or off. Therefore, you are not destined to live out the negative patterns of your forebearers—you can instead make a life choice to overcome by tweaking their patterns of expression. Part 2 of this book will show you how.

Taking this further, the Scriptures that tell us the sins of the parents will reach to the third and fourth generation (Exod. 20:5; 34:7; Num. 14:18) seem to imply that we are responsible for the unconfessed sins of our great-great-grandparents. But we can breathe a sigh of relief when we read Deuteronomy 24:16 and Ezekiel 18:19–20, which explain that we are each responsible for our own sins and not those of our ancestors.

I know this seems confusing, because the Scriptures say that, on the one hand, a parent's iniquity will be visited on the children, but, on the other hand, we are only responsible for our own sins. Here is how it works: Epigenetic changes represent a biological response to an environmental signal. That response can be inherited through the generations via the epigenetic marks. But if you remove the signal, the epigenetic marks will fade.

By the same token, if you choose to add a signal—for example, saying something like, "My mother had depression and that's why I have depression, and now my daughter is suffering from depression"—then the epigenetic marks are activated. The thinking and speaking out the problem serve as the signal that makes it a reality. I have seen this over the years in my private practice and in my seminars, and even in my own life and the lives of my family and friends, time and time again. If we don't wake up to these truths, they will catch us when we are not looking, and before you know it you will be living a life you didn't plan on living. If this is you, here is the good news: You *can* change.

## Predisposition versus Destiny

Herein lies the key: The sins of parents create a *predisposition*, not a *destiny*. You are not responsible for something you are predisposed to because of ancestral decisions. You are responsible, however, to be aware of predispositions, evaluate them, and choose to eliminate them.

The epigenetic marks in our genes that may predispose us to smoke, eat too much of the wrong foods, be negative, or worry can change. This can cause, for example, the genes for obesity to express too strongly or the genes that control stress reactions to switch off, shortening your life as well as decreasing your quality of life and your peace (soul harmony) and happiness. We also are responsible for our own choices and can apply the work of the cross and confess, repent, and eliminate future sinful choices.

In addition, our choices (the epigenetic signals) alter the expression of genes (the epigenetic markers), which can then be passed on to our children and grandchildren, ready to predispose them before they are even conceived. So our bad choices become their bad predispositions.

The negative alternative is that you can choose to accept the predispositions and live into them, but don't forget that you have to take responsibility for that as well. This very act of accepting the predispositions and living into them becomes the signal that activates you to become *a fat and yellow agouti mouse*. Just the addition of a methyl group signal changes the life of the offspring of the agouti mice. In the same way, the addition of a positive attitude signal or a memorized and meditated-upon Scripture signal can change the expression of the gene.

What your mind creates only your mind can take away.

## Scientific Evidence of God's Grace

Another scientific piece of evidence of God's grace can be seen in a structure in the middle of the brain called the *hippocampus*. This seahorse-shaped structure, which processes incoming information, facilitates the conversion of short-term memory to long-term memory, deals with spatial memory, and also helps control our stress response.

Scientists have found that in a loving and nurturing environment, acetyl epigenetic markers increase on the genes in the hippocampus that keep us calm and peaceful. The more acetyl markers, the more these *peace genes* in the hippocampus express and dampen the stress response. A toxic choice produces the opposite effect: The acetyl markers reduce and the methyl markers increase, causing us to have less peace.[4]

So the methyl markers switch off genetic expression and acetyl markers switch on genetic expression. The "switching on or off" is based on the signal, and we can choose to switch. Sometimes we want to switch off—for example switching off the obesity genes in the agouti mice and human research. But we want to switch on good genetic expression—for example the stress control gene in the hippocampus. Whether we switch on happiness, peace, and good health or switch on anxiety, worry, and negativity, we are changing the physical substance of the brain.

## The Brain Reorganizes throughout Our Lifetime

In 1930, Santiago Ramón y Cajal[5] wrote that the nerve pathways are fixed and immutable, but now scientists know that the brain has the amazing ability to reorganize throughout life, changing its structure and function through mental experience alone. If the brain can get worse by constantly focusing on the problem, then the brain can get better by understanding how to eliminate and replace the problem.[6]

# Inside the Brain

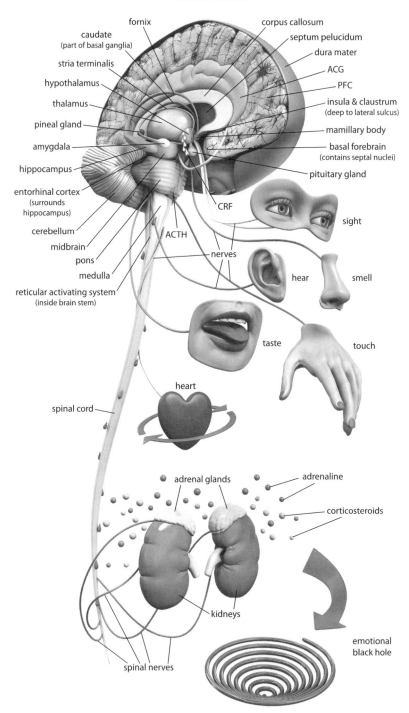

fornix
corpus callosum
caudate (part of basal ganglia)
septum pelucidum
stria terminalis
dura mater
hypothalamus
ACG
thalamus
PFC
pineal gland
insula & claustrum (deep to lateral sulcus)
amygdala
mamillary body
hippocampus
basal forebrain (contains septal nuclei)
entorhinal cortex (surrounds hippocampus)
pituitary gland
cerebellum
CRF
midbrain
sight
pons
ACTH
medulla
nerves
reticular activating system (inside brain stem)
hear
smell
spinal cord
taste
touch
heart
adrenal glands
adrenaline
corticosteroids
kidneys
spinal nerves
emotional black hole

## The Neuroplasticity Paradox

So neuroplasticity can operate for us as well as against us, because whatever we think about the most will grow—this applies to both the positive and negative ends of the spectrum. For example, in post-traumatic stress disorder (PTSD), neuroplasticity has worked against the person. He or she has experienced a crushing mental event that fundamentally changed the meaning of their life and altered the brain structurally because of the neuroplasticity of the brain. During the trauma, the person's mind was not thinking in soul harmony (Col. 3:15 AMP), so consequently he or she did not choose, process, or react correctly to the event—making the thought that became wired in a jumbled toxic mess. As the person relives the event over and over, it wires itself deeper into the mind, becoming a main filter and disrupting normal function.[7] Flashbacks—reliving the bad memory many times a day—strengthen the circuit, making it worse and more debilitating.

## We Can Use Neuroplasticity to Renew Our Minds

How do we fix this? In part 2, I will explain this in depth and supply a simple explanation and a chart of my theory in chapter 8, "The Geodesic Information Processing Theory,"[8] upon which my approach is based. The overriding concept is to apply neuroplasticity in the correct direction by rewiring the event with the positive thinking of Philippians 4:8: "Finally, brothers, whatever is true, whatever is honorable, whatever is just, whatever is pure, whatever is lovely, whatever is commendable, if there is any excellence, if there is anything worthy of praise, think about these things" (ESV).

Thus the person consciously chooses, preferably under the leading of the Holy Spirit, to bring the memory into consciousness where it becomes plastic enough to actually be changed.

This means the physical substrate of the memory becomes weakened, vulnerable, malleable, and able to be manipulated. The person then chooses to replace the crushing mental event with the implanted word of God, which saves the soul (James 1:21). The person, as though an outsider looking in through a window, will observe the toxic, traumatic memory as a weakening and dying experience but, at the same time, observe the new healthy experience that is growing. In practicing this daily, the person wires the healthy new thoughts ever more deeply into the mind.

Neurons that don't get enough signal (the rehearsing of the negative event) will start firing apart, wiring apart, pulling out, and destroying the emotion attached to the trauma. In addition, certain chemicals like oxytocin (bonds and remolds chemicals), dopamine (increases focus and attention), and serotonin (increases feelings of peace and happiness) all start flowing around the traumatic thoughts, weakening them even more. This all helps to disconnect and desynchronize the neurons; if they stop firing together, they will no longer wire together. This leads to wiping out or popping those connections and rebuilding new ones. I explain the practical side of this process in part 2.

## More Encouragement from Science

There are even more encouraging pieces of information about neuroplasticity. For example, Universalists believe logic and language are learned at fixed ages, and if you pass that fixed age, you can't learn. Plasticity research proves them wrong.[9] People with learning disabilities can rewire their brains to perceive sound better.[10] My own patients with brain injuries and learning and emotional disabilities, as well as the teachers and students I have worked with in schools, showed significant changes when they did the mental training in my Switch On Your Brain technique.[11]

The media creates incorrect perceptions of scientific discoveries. They may cover a study that sensationalizes that our brain does x, therefore you will do x, as though you cannot think for yourself. This is so wrong. Those who believe you are just your brain believe you have no free will. The active mind changes the brain; the brain is the passive part of existence. As we think, we are making the brain fire in different patterns and combinations, and whenever we make the brain fire differently, we change the brain. Epigenetics research demonstrates that our lifestyles and environment can transform the way our genes are expressed, and evidence from this field shows us we are not being controlled by the structure of our brains.[12]

One brain generates more energy (electrical impulses) in one day than all the cell phones on the planet.[13] So we have the power to make changes; we do not have a spirit of fear, but of love, power, and a sound mind (see 2 Tim. 1:7). Our default mind mode—our soul, which is our intellect, will, and emotions—is powerful, strong, and driven by principles of love. Don't let the media, doctors, or other people in your life convince you otherwise. You have the power in your mind to change the negative, toxic manifestations. Our minds shape the world. This is what neuroplasticity is all about: change. Neuroplasticity is God's design for renewing the mind.

## Our Perceptions Count

Our perception of the environment plus how we manage our environment controls our bodies and lives. So if you change your perception, you change your biology. You become the master of your life instead of a victim. But don't do it without Christ; remember, he is the vine from which we grow (John 15:5). The billion-dollar self-help industry does not have sustainability[14] because it misses the basic elements required for success and change: Primarily, it is not connected to the vine. These practitioners try to teach successful living without the originator of successful living: God. Secondly, there is a lot of visualization and verbalizations in their advice, but the intent of the heart is not considered, leaving a disconnect between what is being said and what is really believed and felt deep down. This is called cognitive dissonance. Thirdly, there is often very little real action involved. Action on both a spiritual and scientific level is required for change to take place.

Research also shows that there is a negative side to positive self-statements and affirmations, showing that individuals with low self-esteem felt worse after repeating positive self-statements.[15] Don't become part of that statistic.

The world may tell us that the mind is what the brain does, but God tells us that the brain will do what the mind tells it to do. And when your spirit, under the leading of the Holy Spirit, controls your soul, then the gold standard of thinking is achieved. This is a very different perspective from the traditional view, which tells us we are machines that just need parts changed and chemicals added. Choices are real; you are free to make choices about how you focus your attention, and this affects how the chemicals and wiring of your brain change and function.

Scientists are now proving that the relationship between you and how you understand and perceive your inner thought life, your community, and God has a huge impact on how your brain works.[16] Moment by moment of each day you can choose who you will be in the next moment, and these choices are captured in the resultant thought networks you build. In that process, the precepts of Scripture should be the overarching, undergirding, and foundational framework. They should be so entrenched that our attention is viewed through them and them alone as we form a view of ourselves that God created us to be.

Personally, my spiritual life informs my scientific life. As Joshua 1:8 says, insight, mindfulness, and wisdom come through meditation on God's truth versus rote study of information. I want to shape my world around God's truth because I know as a scientist and a believer, paying attention to my thoughts and purposefully focusing my mind leads to great transformations.

## You Have the Power to Change

Your patterns of genetic experience don't determine what you are; you do. How you live, the cultural environment you live in, whatever you immerse yourself in, your beliefs and the beliefs of those around you, how you interact with those people, your faith and how you grow it, what you expose yourself to—all of these lead to differences in the way you focus your attention and have a direct effect on how your proteins are synthesized, how your enzymes act, and how your neurochemicals work together. If you don't believe you have the power to change your thoughts and control your choices, you are not going to do it.

Doing your own brain surgery or neuroplastic intervention of toxic thinking and renewing your mind is based on regular exercising of your brain; change takes place over time through continual persistence. Intervention of the mind changes the brain physically, chemically, structurally, and functionally. Research shows there is no more effective way to produce localized and specific changes in the brain than behavioral or mental intervention. Since psychosocial factors modulate the course of certain diseases—such as cardiovascular disease, diabetes, and asthma—this means the things going on in the environment get into the mind, changing the brain and having an impact on the body. So it is vital for us to pay attention to the precepts laid down in God's Word. Understanding how God designed neuroplasticity to work for and against us will help us move forward.

## Chapter 3 Summary

1. Our thoughts, imagination, and choices can change the structure and function of our brains on every level: molecular, genetic, epigenetic, cellular, structural, neurochemical, and electromagnetic, and even subatomic. Through our thoughts, we can be our own brain surgeons as we make choices that change the circuits in our brain. We are designed to do our own brain surgery.

2. Choices become signals that change our brain and body, and these changes are not necessarily dictated by our genes.

3. Epigenetics is referred to as a new science, but actually it is an ancient science that we find throughout the Bible. At its most basic level, epigenetics is the fact that your thoughts and choices impact your physical brain and body, your mental health, and your spiritual development.

4. These choices will affect not only your *own* spirit, soul, and body but also the people with whom you have

relationships. In fact, it goes even deeper: Your choices might impact the generations that follow.

5. The landmark study on agouti mice fostered a host of studies—including some done on humans—that show that not only does food change generational patterns, but so does thinking.

6. Taken collectively, these studies show us that the good, the bad, and the ugly do come down through the generations. But your mind is the signal—the epigenetic factor—that switches these genes on or off.

7. Therefore, you are not destined to live out the negative patterns of your forebearers, but you can instead make a life choice to overcome them by tweaking their expression. In part 2 of this book I will show you how.

8. Epigenetic changes represent a biological response to an environmental signal. That response can be inherited through the generations via the epigenetic marks. But if you remove the signal, the epigenetic marks will fade. If you choose to add a signal, then the epigenetic marks are activated.

9. Herein lies the key: The sins of parents can create a *predisposition*, not a *destiny*. You are not responsible for something you are predisposed to because of ancestral decisions. You are responsible, however, to be aware of them, evaluate those predispositions, and choose to eliminate them.

10. When you make a bad choice, genes switch on in the hippocampus that dampen the stress response.

11. Scientists now know that the brain has the amazing ability to reorganize throughout life, changing its structure and function through thinking alone.

12. Neuroplasticity (the ability of the brain to change in response to thinking) can operate for you as well as against you because whatever you think about the most will grow. This applies to both the positive and negative ends of the spectrum.

13. Our perception of the environment plus how we manage our environment controls our bodies and lives. So if you change your perception, you change your biology. You become the master of your life instead of a victim.

# 4

# Catch Those Thoughts

> **Main Scripture:** We destroy arguments and every lofty opinion raised against the knowledge of God, and take every thought captive to obey Christ. 2 Corinthians 10:5 ESV
>
> **Linked Science Concept:** When you objectively observe your own thinking with the view to capturing rogue thoughts, you in effect direct your attention to stop the negative impact and rewire healthy new circuits into your brain.

The ability to quiet your mind, focus your attention on the present issue, capture your thoughts, and dismiss the distractions that come your way is an excellent and powerful ability that God has placed within you. In the busy age we live in, however, we have trained ourselves out of this natural and necessary skill. *Natural* because it is wired into the design of the brain, allowing the brain to capture and discipline chaotic rogue thoughts; *necessary* because it calms our spirits so we can tune in and listen to God. When we are mindful of catching our thoughts in this way, we change our connection with God from uninvolved and independent to involved and dependent.

Research dating back to the 1970s shows that capturing our thoughts in a disciplined way rather than letting them chaotically run rampant can bring about impressive changes in how we feel and think. This change is evidenced in cognitive, emotional functioning as well as at the neural level.[1] My research shows that controlled focused thinking leads to impressive improvement in cognitive functioning and emotional balance.[2]

## Freeing Yourself from Burdens

Getting your thoughts disciplined and under control is one of the first steps in freeing yourself of the burdens of the world and beginning to enjoy life despite the burdens of the world.

When you objectively observe your own thinking with the view to capturing rogue thoughts, you in effect direct your attention to stop the negative impact and rewire healthy new circuits into your brain. Second Corinthians 10:3–5 is so clear in the instructions on this matter: "For though we live in the world, we do not wage war as the world does. The weapons we fight with are not the weapons of the world. On the contrary, they have divine power to demolish strongholds. We demolish arguments and every pretension that sets itself up against the knowledge of God, and we take captive every thought to make it obedient to Christ" (NIV). In Proverbs 4:20–22 the sage advice is to "give attention to my words; incline your ear to my sayings. Do not let them depart from your eyes; keep them in the midst of your heart; for they are life to those who find them, and health to all their flesh."

The primary success of capturing your thoughts will be to focus on God's way first, not the world's ways. And science is showing that meditating on the elements of Jesus's teachings rewires healthy new circuits in the brain.

## Science Shows the Benefits of Catching Your Thoughts

When you make a conscious decision to focus and direct your attention correctly, you change physical matter—your brain and your body change in a healthy way. Purposefully catching your thoughts can control the brain's sensory processing, the brain's rewiring, the neurotransmitters, the genetic expression, and cellular activity in a positive or negative direction. You choose.

The benefits are even greater than the scientists back in the '70s and '80s imagined. My patients who were successful in therapy took their first steps to success when they started focusing their attention and capturing their thoughts—for example "I can't do this," "It's too hard," "It's never worked before," and "I am not smart enough." The benefits of catching any negative thoughts like these cannot be emphasized enough. Not catching those thoughts will lead to a potential spiral into confusion and varying levels of mental despair.

## Dr. Jekyll and Mr. Hyde

An interesting body of research shows how a certain type of protein, called a "prion protein," operates a bit like a Dr. Jekyll and Mr. Hyde—the story often used as a metaphor of the good man who hides an evil side. When a prion protein folds over itself, it plays a crucial role in neurodegenerative diseases that lead to dreadful syndromes such as the mad cow disease. But scientists have now found that the prion protein abounds in synapses—the contact point where signals are passed from one nerve cell to the next. Prions help create long-term, self-sustaining memories. They are also important in neuroplasticity, which is the change and rewiring that happens in our brain when we think and learn; and finally, they are involved in neurogenesis.[3] The point here is that this protein does amazing things in the brain in response to good signals and goes crazy in response to negative signals. A chaotic mind filled with uncaptured rogue thoughts of anxiety, worry, and any and all manner of fear-related emotions sends out the wrong signal.

## Another Example of a Vicious Cycle

Stress is the key to understanding the association between depression and heart disease. Research shows that 40 to 60 percent of heart disease patients suffer clinical depression and 30 to 50 percent of patients who suffer clinical depression are at risk for heart disease.[4]

Not catching and stopping those thoughts leads to negative, toxic thoughts being wired into the brain; this can lead to depressive thoughts, which causes the body to go into stage two of stress. In response, the immune system produces proteins called *cytokines*, including one called *Interleukin-6*, as a positive, inflammatory response to protect the brain and body against stress. If the stress is not controlled, the depression increases and the person moves into stress stage 3; over time the inflammation also increases and can lead to arteriosclerosis (hardening of the arteries) and cardiovascular disease.

All this is from not catching those negative, toxic thoughts. And this is just one disease process; there are a multitude of other manifestations of not stopping this cycle. Recent research has shown that teaching strategies to handle and control stress (the body's reaction to toxic thinking) could make individuals who are vulnerable to schizophrenia and other neuropsychiatric disorders less vulnerable.[5]

## It Only Takes Five to Sixteen Minutes a Day

Research has shown that five to sixteen minutes a day of focused, meditative capturing of thoughts shifts frontal brain states that are more likely to engage with the world.[6] Research also showed that those same five to sixteen minutes of intense, deep thinking activity increased the chances of a happier outlook on life.

God has blessed us with powerful and sound minds (2 Tim. 2:17). When we direct our attention by capturing our thoughts, we provide a target for our mental faculties. Then God will give you a project and your balance will be restored. If you don't let God give you a thinking project, the Enemy will surely step in to try to catch your thoughts and destroy your balance.

God has designed the frontal lobe of our brains precisely to do this: handle his thought projects. This perspective is highlighted in the Message version of 2 Corinthians 10:5: "We use our powerful God-tools for smashing warped philosophies, tearing down barriers erected against the truth of God, fitting every loose thought and emotion and impulse into the structure of life shaped by Christ. Our tools are ready at hand for clearing the ground of every obstruction and building lives of obedience into maturity."

## Our Normal Is Perfection

Because we are made in God's image (Gen. 1:26) and have the "mind of Christ" (1 Cor. 2:16), our normal state is one of perfection.

Science now is able to demonstrate that we are "wired for love," and fear, which incorporates anything toxic, is therefore not our norm. This means our natural fashioned-after-God inclination is one of optimism and good, healthy thinking. We therefore have a God-given freedom to choose right or wrong—but it comes with conditions attached: "I have set before you life and death, blessing and cursing; therefore choose life, that both you and your descendants may live" (Deut. 30:19). This is clearly evidenced in the brain—when bad choices are made, or those negative thoughts are not captured, the neural wiring becomes distorted, which results in disruption of normal function.

God designed humans to observe our own thoughts, catch those that are bad, and get rid of them. The importance of capturing those thoughts cannot be underestimated because research shows that the vast majority of mental and physical illness comes from our thought life rather than the environment and genes.[7]

An undisciplined mind is filled with a continuous stream of worries, fears, and distorted perceptions that trigger degenerative processes in the mind and body. We cannot afford not to bring all thoughts into captivity to Christ Jesus (2 Cor. 10:5).

## Chapter 4 Summary

1. The design of the brain allows us to capture and discipline chaotic thoughts.
2. Catching our thoughts is *necessary* because it calms our spirits so we can tune in and listen to God.
3. When we are mindful of catching our thoughts in this way, we change our connection with God from uninvolved and independent to involved and dependent.

4. Research dating back to the 1970s shows that being introspectively aware of our thoughts in a disciplined way rather than letting them chaotically run rampant can bring about impressive changes in how we feel and think.

5. Purposefully catching your thoughts can control the brain's sensory processing, the brain's rewiring, the neurotransmitters, the genetic expression, and cellular activity in a positive or negative direction. You choose.

6. A chaotic mind filled with uncaptured rogue thoughts of anxiety, worry, and all manner of fear-related emotions sends out the wrong signal right down to the level of the DNA.

7. Research has shown that five to sixteen minutes a day of focused, meditative capturing of thoughts shifts frontal brain states so that they are more likely to engage with the world and increases the chances of a happier outlook on life.

8. We are wired for love and then learn fear.

# 5

# Entering into Directed Rest

**Main Scripture:** Be still, and know that I am God. Psalm 46:10

**Linked Science Concept:** When we direct our rest by introspection, self-reflection, and prayer; when we catch our thoughts; when we memorize and quote Scripture; and when we develop our mind intellectually, we enhance the default mode network (DMN) that improves brain function and mental, physical, and spiritual health.

God's order is clearly reflected in the organization of the brain. God has designed the brain to work in a series of coordinated networks. The scientific expression for this is *integrative functional organization*, which basically means that all parts of the brain are connected, work together, and impact each other.

God has also designed the brain in such a way that the intrinsic activity in the nonconscious part of our minds is where most of the *mind-action* takes place, and it is always dominant, twenty-four hours a day. It is where we are think-ing, choosing, building, and sorting thoughts. Simply put, it is the constant, high-energy activity that is always going on in the nonconscious mind, even when we are resting. What we consciously think and what we say and do is all driven by the information and activity in the nonconscious mind. So the nonconscious mind has the roots of all our words and ac-tions, and we choose with our minds what these roots will be.

This organizational structure of the brain and body is described in Ephesians 4:16: "He makes the whole body fit together perfectly. As each part does its own special work, it helps the other parts grow, so that the whole body is healthy and growing and full of love" (NLT).

The constant, high-intrinsic activity in the brain that influ-ences our words and actions can be seen in the Scriptures: "As he thinks in his heart, so is he" (Prov. 23:7).

What research shows is that when we go into a directed rest—a focused, introspective state—we enhance and increase the effectiveness of the activity in the nonconscious. Research shows that there is a greater increase in gamma waves, which are involved in attention, memory building, and learning, and more activity linked to positive emotions like happiness when we move into this directed rest state. PET scans and EEG recordings show portions of the brain bulk up that produce happiness and peace.[1] This is wisdom from Psalm 46:10: "Be still, and know that I am God."

## The Organized Networks in the Brain

Let's take a closer look at these coordinated and organized networks in our brains that work together in a busy, integrated, and balanced way, helping our brains maintain a high level of activity 24/7. These networks form the brain's inner life with the default mode network (DMN) dominating and becoming especially active when the mind is introspective and thinking deeply in a directed rest or idling state.

The DMN acts much like the conductor of an orchestra giving timing signals and coordinating activity among the different brain networks and regions and getting the brain ready to react on a conscious level. For example, the DMN coordinates the activity in

- networks that become active during a mental task;
- networks that are active during memory formation and when we pay attention;
- the salience network, which helps determine what we pay attention to; and
- the sensory-motor network, which integrates the brain's control of body movements with sensory feedback.

When your mind is busy with intrinsic activity (which is basically directed rest) such as introspection and thinking things through, letting your mind wander, sleeping, deep thinking, even under anesthetic, there is a constant chatter between the networks of the brain in the nonconscious mind. The energy consumed by this constantly active messaging and thought building in the nonconscious level of our mind is about twenty times more than when we are conscious. When we move into an alert conscious state, the energy consumption in the brain increases by 5 percent. In fact, 60 to 80 percent of all energy used by the brain occurs in circuits inside the brain that are unrelated to any external signal. This is all predominant DMN activity.[2]

## Flexibility

An important property of these brain networks is called *anti-correlation*, which means we switch back and forth between the various networks.[3] For example, when we have flexible and creative thinking, we are able to shift between thoughts and capture and control thoughts. This is good and is what we want.

We need this flexibility as we go through life. We cannot control the events and circumstances of life, but we can control our *reactions* to those events and circumstances. Controlling our reactions requires flexibility in our thinking, and God has given us that with our multiple, different networks. God has designed our brain to work for us and not to control us.

## Switch Off to Switch On

What I find fascinating is that when we shift into the default mode network (DMN), we don't switch off to rest. Quite the contrary, we *switch off to switch on* to a mode of thinking that gives us perspective and wisdom and the opportunity to connect with God. This is a state of mind in which we switch off to the external and switch on to the internal.

In this deeply intellectual state, involved networks remain active, and the shifting between them remains active, but it is a different kind of activity. It is more focused and introspective. So when our brain enters the rest circuit, we don't actually rest; we move into a highly intelligent, self-reflective, directed state. And the more often we go there, the more we get in touch with the deep, spiritual part of who we are. I believe God has created this state to directly connect us to him and to develop and practice an awareness of his presence. As the Scripture says, "Keep awake (give strict attention, be cautious and active) and watch and pray, that you may not come into temptation. The spirit indeed is willing, but the flesh is weak" (Matt. 26:41 AMP).

The DMN is a primary network that we switch into when we switch off from the outside world and move into a state of focused mindfulness. It activates to even higher levels when a person is daydreaming, introspecting, or letting his or her mind wander in an organized exploratory way through the endless myriad of thoughts within the mind. It's a directed, deeply intellectual focusing inward and tuning out the outside world. It is a cessation from active external, which is like the Sabbath when we switch off from the world and focus on God.

In this directed rest state, you focus inward, you introspect, and you appear to slow down; but actually, your mental resources speed up and your thinking moves onto a higher level. When you think in this way, when you pause your activity and enter into a directed rest, you will emerge far ahead of where you would have been if you just operated within the realms of a shifting, shuffling, limited conscious, cognitive mind. This is the state of being still and knowing that he is God (Ps. 46:10).

The DMN, which used to be thought of as *dark energy* in the brain, is activated into ever-higher states when we engage in self-referential activity. Brain imaging experiments show that there is a persistent level of background activity when a person is in a state of directed rest.[4] This includes recollections, ruminations, imaginations, and self-perceptions; and it involves the ability to focus on a specific memory, thinking through things from different angles while still being solution focused. It is very important in planning future actions.[5]

In fact, miswiring of brain regions involved in the DMN, leading to all kinds of ups and downs in the DMN, may even be part of disorders ranging from Alzheimer's to schizophrenia to other neuropsychiatric disorders. Research is starting to show that, for example, brain areas that atrophy and die in Alzheimer's overlap with major centers of the DMN. Patients with depression show decreased connectivity between certain regions of the DMN and the emotional areas of the brain. And in schizophrenia, many areas of the DMN showed increased activity levels.[6]

Regular meditators—by this I mean those who have adopted a disciplined and focused, reflecting thought life in which they bring all thoughts into captivity—show that their DMN is more active and that there is more switching back and forth between networks.[7] This means the brain is more active, growing more branches and integrating and linking thoughts, which translates as increased intelligence and wisdom and that wonderful feeling of peace. God also throws in some additional benefits such as increased immune and cardiovascular health.

When we pray, when we catch our thoughts, when we memorize and quote Scripture, we move into this deep meditative state. This great state of mind is also activated when we intellectualize deeply about information—perhaps what we are studying or a skill we are developing in our job. We are highly intellectual beings created to have relationship with a highly intellectual God. We should never underestimate how brilliant we are and that we are only limited by how we see ourselves.

## In His Great Mercy

In his great mercy, God has wired into the design of our brain these circuits that are spearheaded by the default mode network (DMN) we need to regularly access to keep connected to our spirits and to be able to follow the leading of the Holy Spirit—a time of ceasing from our own activity, ceasing from our own efforts (Heb. 4:9–10). Our minds need time to understand what our spirits already know.

In the busyness of life and the flurry of everyday activity, we expose ourselves to the possibility of developing a chaotic mindset with the net result of neurochemical and electromagnetic chaos in the brain. This feels like endless loops and spirals of thinking that can easily get out of control. When we activate the DMN, however, it is almost like a Sabbath in the brain, which is a cessation from the conscious flurry of work and a withdrawal into the depths of our mind. It is like a mental rebooting process to reconnect with who we are and with our Savior to bring perspective to the issues of life.

## The Sabbath in the Brain

In fact, when we don't frequently slow down and enter this rest state, this *Sabbath* in the brain, we disrupt natural functions in the brain. Research shows that when we don't engage in this disciplined and focused self-reflective pattern of thinking that activates the DMN, we may experience negative self-esteem, depression, worry, anxiety, and health issues, and over-focus on generalized and short-term memory issues. We may get stuck, unable to cope, and have a tendency to focus on the problem and not the solution. In fact, as things go wrong in the processing of information in the default mode network, the mishandled data is passed on to other networks in the brain where it creates additional problems.[8] These additional problems can be experienced as memory issues, cloudy and fuzzy thinking, anxiety, depression, and many other manifestations including neuropsychiatric disorders.

## The Task Positive Network

In line with the amazing order and balance God created in everything, we find this default mode resting network is balanced by the task positive network (TPN). The TPN supports the active thinking required for making decisions.[9] So as we focus our thinking and activate the DMN, at some point in our thinking process we move into active decision-making. This activates the TPN, and we experience this as action. In my 21-Day Brain Detox Plan (discussed in part 2), I call this action an *active reach*. Brain research—specifically the science of thought[10]—shows that action completes the cycle of building up and breaking down thoughts. We see this in the Scriptures as well: "Faith without works is dead" (James 2:26).

What is very interesting, and sobering, however, is how our DMN and TPN networks, as well as the balance between the two, are thrown off when we choose to be toxic. Toxic negative thinking produces increased activity in the DMN, and activity in the TPN decreases. This results in maladaptive, depressive ruminations and a decrease in the ability to solve problems. This makes us feel foggy, confused, negative, and depressed.

God is a God of order and balance, and he has fashioned our spirit, soul, and body this way. So it is quite simple; when we don't follow his ordinances, there will be consequences. The brain moves into an unbalanced state, producing neurochemical and electromagnetic chaos. "For where you have envy and selfish ambition, there you find disorder and every evil practice" (James 3:16 NIV).

## Our Brain Follows Our Mind

Studies using imaging techniques show that the DMN activates abnormally in individuals with depression.[11] Other studies show that in depressed individuals, the front middle part of the brain (anterior medial cortex) has increased activity.[12] This means that although their ruminations increased, this good sign was thrown into disarray by decreased activity in the middle-back part of the brain (the posterior medial cortex). When there is decreased activity in the posterior medial cortex, a pattern of dissociation occurs and there is a tendency to move away from being clear and specific in thinking about memories toward focusing on overly general memories.[13]

What this means is that when rumination turns into unproductive brooding and negative issues are blown out of proportion, it is detrimental to the brain and to good life choices. When this happens, healthy focused introspection activating the DMN turns from a coping-and-solution focus to a passive-and-maladaptive focus, which can result in worrying, anxiety, and depression.

This gives us scientific proof that we need to have the mindset expressed in Philippians 4:8: "Finally, brothers and sisters, whatever is true, whatever is noble, whatever is right, whatever is pure, whatever is lovely, whatever is admirable—if anything is excellent or praiseworthy—think about such things" (NIV). By following this perfect advice from God's Word, you can bring back the balance between the default mode network (DMN) and the task positive network (TPN).

## The Seven Different Types of Thinking

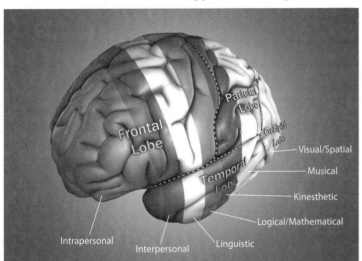

The good news is that this balance can be restored very quickly when you choose to become introspective and ruminate in a positive, directed way.[14] The speed of the change in how you feel and function is not just because of the balance being restored between the DMN and TPN, but also because the brain functions in complex circuits that encompass multiple brain structures and regions, so there is a positive, cascading effect throughout the brain. This is, once again, God's grace in action.

### Consequences of Toxic Thinking

Throughout this book, the resounding message is that negative thinking creates atypical responses in the brain, which will result in atypical manifestations. Studies have clearly demonstrated that people with a history of various types of depression exhibit differences in the regions and circuits of the brain associated with knowledge of socially acceptable behavior (anterior temporal lobe) and the awareness of wrong (subgenual region of the brain).[15]

Their thoughts and the choices they have made changed their brain in a negative way so that instead of being convicted of wrong in order to change—which is positive—they felt guilty and condemned, causing the positive to become negative.[16]

Other studies dealing with obsessive compulsive disorders[17] and schizophrenia[18] show definite changes in the brain from the negative to the positive when thinking is brought under control. Some scientists even describe these neuropsychiatric manifestations almost as though negative, toxic thinking opens a gate that allows negative emotions to overwhelm them. And because mind changes matter, this negative thinking changes the brain structure.

Patients with schizophrenia have decreased activity between their thalamus and prefrontal cortex, which affects memory and behavioral flexibility. They also have incorrect activity in their decision-making and emotional areas of the brain. From studies of adolescents starting to show symptoms of schizophrenia, it appears the areas are overactive at first from toxic stress reactions and then become damaged and hypoactive. So if we don't help our children and adolescents manage stress, we are potentially causing brain damage, which in turn leads to more serious problems.[19]

Other research shows that women who have suffered abuse were 60 percent more likely to have a child with autism. The researchers propose that the long-lasting effects of abuse on women's biological systems, such as the immune system and stress-response system, are responsible for increasing their likelihood of having a child with autism.[20] These women were victims of toxic thinking and the stress it causes—and the abuse will therefore impact the next generation as well, and potentially the next three. This is why there are often family histories of autism. I tell you this study to highlight the responsibility we have in not only getting our own minds right but also helping others, especially victims of trauma, get their minds right.

## Switch On Your Brain

Choosing to be focused and mindful and to activate your DMN and your TPN in a balanced way by capturing your thoughts will bring you back in alignment with God.

In my 21-Day Brain Detox Plan, I show you how to center your attention on a single element, using my Switch On Your Brain 5-Step Learning Process. When there is a pause in your activity, a quiet state, that is a perfect time to connect to the spiritual part of who you are. In this state your mind can begin to understand what your spirit knows. You can position yourself to let the Holy Spirit deposit truth and direction in your spirit as you "trust in the LORD with all your heart, and lean not on your own understanding; in all your ways acknowledge Him, and He shall direct your paths" (Prov. 3:5–6).

Through modifying our practices of thought toward a more disciplined, focused, and reflective thought life, we can build up healthy neural *real estate* that is better able to bring our thoughts into captivity and deal with the variegated demands of today's modern world. Your mind can powerfully and unexpectedly change your brain in positive ways when you intentionally direct your attention. The most efficient way to improve your brain is a daily step-by-step process— a lifestyle of thinking your brain into better functioning so that it turns into whatever *you* expect it to be: "As he thinks in his heart, so is he" (Prov. 23:7).

Your mind, intellect, will, and emotions are always changing your brain in some way. Directed, disciplined, and focused attention on the correct things is a major key to switching on your brain.

## Chapter 5 Summary

1. We have all kinds of coordinated networks in our brains that work together in an organized way, forming a constant, intrinsic *chatter* in the nonconscious part of our mind.

2. Our brains maintain a high level of activity 24/7. This activity forms the brain's inner life, with the default mode network (DMN) dominating and becoming especially active when the mind is introspective and thinking deeply in a directed rest or idle state.

3. As these networks function correctly, we shift into deeply introspective and meditative states that increase our intelligence and health.

4. When we switch back and forth between the various networks—for example, when we have flexible and creative thinking—we are able to shift between thoughts and capture and control them.

5. When we direct our rest by introspection, self-reflection, and prayer; when we catch our thoughts; when we memorize and quote Scripture; when we develop our mind intellectually, we accelerate the default mode network (DMN) and improve brain function as well as mind, body, and spiritual health.

6. The DMN is balanced by the task positive network (TPN), which supports the active thinking required for making decisions. The more balanced we are, the more wisdom we apply in our thinking and decisions. This action step of the TPN is necessary for effective mind and brain change.

7. Miswiring of brain regions involved in the DMN that leads to all kinds of ups and downs in the DMN may even be part of disorders ranging from Alzheimer's to schizophrenia.

8. Toxic thinking produces this miswiring, which causes increased activity in the DMN, resulting in a decrease of activity in the TPN. This causes maladaptive, depressive ruminations and a decrease in the ability to solve problems. This makes us feel foggy, confused, negative, and depressed.

9. Your mind can powerfully and unexpectedly change your brain in positive ways when you intentionally direct your attention.

# 6

# Stop Milkshake-Multitasking

**Main Scripture:** Dear friend, listen well to my words; tune your ears to my voice. Keep my message in plain view at all times. Concentrate! Learn it by heart! Those who discover these words live, really live; body and soul, they're bursting with health. Keep vigilant watch over your heart; that's where life starts. Proverbs 4:20–23 Message

**Linked Science Concept:** Multitasking is a persistent myth. Paying deep, focused attention to one task at a time is the correct way.

One of the plagues of modern existence is multitasking, which leads to the further plagues of "hurry sickness" and obsessive time management. The truth about multitasking is that it is a persistent myth. What we really do is shift our attention rapidly from task to task, resulting in two bad things: (1) We don't devote as much focused attention as we should to a specific activity, task, or piece of information, and (2) we sacrifice the quality of our attention. I call this "milkshake-multitasking."

## Multitasking Is a Persistent Myth

This poor focusing of attention and lack of quality in our thought lives is the complete opposite of how the brain is designed to function and causes a level of brain damage. Every rapid, incomplete, and poor quality shift of thought is like making a milkshake with your brain cells and neurochemicals. This milkshake-multitasking, which is the truth behind multitasking, creates patterns of flightiness and lack of concentration that are unfortunately often erroneously labeled ADD and ADHD and that are too often unnecessarily medicated, adding fuel to the fire. And it's a rapid downhill slide from there if we don't get back to our God-design of deep, intellectual attention.

What does deep, focused, intellectual attention look like versus milkshake-multitasking? The answer is modeled in Proverbs 4:20–23: "Dear friend, listen well to my words; tune your ears to my voice. Keep my message in plain view at all times. Concentrate! Learn it by heart! Those who discover these words live, really live; body and soul, they're bursting with health. Keep vigilant watch over your heart; that's where life starts" (Message). It is very interesting that every cell in the body is connected to the heart, and the brain controls the heart and the mind controls the brain. So whatever we are thinking about affects every cell in our body.

We saw in the last chapter that we are deeply intellectual beings and are designed to bring all thoughts into captivity— are you surprised? We are made in God's image, after all. He designed us to think through things one at a time in a focused, quality manner by paying attention, listening intently, keeping our eyes on one thing at a time, and fixing it in our mind.

## The 140-Character Tweet

This design described above contrasts undeniably with the general pattern of modern life today in which so much attention is paid to tweeting on Twitter, Instagramming, and Facebooking to the point that we forget all about enjoying the moment. We are told by so-called social media experts that information needs to be in bite-size amounts and in a constant stream of new information before the previous information has even been digested.

This is not stimulation; it is bombardment. We have been reduced to 140 characters and an addiction to looking for the next informational high. Students can't sit quietly and enjoy reading a book, allowing their imagination to take flight.

Before sharing some of the researched consequences of this milkshake-multitasking momentum we are in, I want to assure you that I believe social media plays an important role in society, business, and life. When used correctly and in a balanced way, it is a phenomenal communications tool. I am all for progress. Used incorrectly, however, this good thing becomes a bad thing.

## It's All about Balance

It is all about balance. Our brain responds with healthy patterns, circuits, and neurochemicals when we think deeply, but not when we skim only the surface of multiple pieces of information. Colossians 3:15 in the Amplified Bible explains peace as "soul harmony" that comes from Christ and that acts as an umpire who helps us think, choose, decide, and settle with finality all questions that arise in our minds. But milkshake-multitasking switches on confusion in our brain, making soul harmony impossible.

Scientists have found that the amount of time spent milkshake-multitasking among American young people has increased by 120 percent in the last ten years. According to a report in the *Archives of General Psychiatry*, simultaneous exposure to electronic media during the teenage years—such as playing a computer game while watching television—appears to be associated with increased depression and anxiety in young adulthood, especially among men.[1] Considering that teens are exposed to an average of eight and a half hours of multitasking electronic media per day, we need to change something quickly.[2]

## Social Media Enthusiast or Addict?

Another concern this raises is whether you are or your teen is a social media enthusiast or simply a social media addict? This is a very real problem—so much so that researchers from Norway developed a new instrument to measure Facebook addiction called the Bergen Facebook Addiction Scale.[3] Social media has become as ubiquitous as television in our everyday lives, and this research shows that multitasking social media can be as addictive as drugs, alcohol, and chemical substance abuse.

A large number of friends on social media networks may appear impressive, but according to a new report, the more social circles a person is linked to, the more likely the social media will be a source of stress.[4] It can also have a detrimental effect on consumer well-being because milkshake-multitasking interferes with clear thinking and decision-making, which lowers self-control and leads to rash, impulsive buying and poor eating decisions. Greater social media use is associated with a higher body mass index, increased binge eating, a lower credit score, and higher levels of credit card debt for consumers with many close friends in their social network— all caused by a lack of self-control.[5]

## We Can Become Shallow

Milkshake-multitasking decreases our attention, making us increasingly less able to focus on our thought habits. This opens us up to shallow and weak judgments and decisions and results in passive mindlessness. Deep, intellectual thought, however, results in interactive mindfulness—the "soul harmony" presented in Colossians 3:15 (AMP). This requires engaging passionately with the world. We need to increase our awareness of our thoughts and take the time to understand and reflect on them.

Let's take a look at some studies that show the impact of changing from a milkshake-multitasking mindset to a deep, intellectual mindset.

In 2012 a research group at the University of Washington did an interesting study on the effects of meditation training on multitasking. They found that the subjects of the study had fewer negative emotions, could stay on task longer, had improved concentration, switched between tasks more effectively in a focused and organized way, as opposed to haphazardly dashing back and forth between tasks, and spent their time more efficiently.[6] These results excited me because I found similar results in my own research.[7]

## My Research

In my documented research with patients who had traumatic brain injury (TBI) and students and adults who had learning and emotional disabilities, I was astounded at the change in their cognitive and emotional function once they started applying a more deeply intellectual thinking pattern. I abandoned all traditional therapy, trained them in a new technique I had developed, and showed them how to apply it to their daily life. The changes were almost immediate: improved focus, concentration, understanding, shifting efficiency, and overall effectiveness in producing quality work. There were even positive emotional changes, specifically in self-motivation and self-esteem. And it didn't stop there; over time they continued to improve in cognitive and emotional functioning. Once they were set on a healthy thinking path, it continued upward in a cascading fashion.

In the ensuing past twenty years, I have seen these improvements in thousands of patients and clients. This work is the result of God's guidance, because when I started down this path, it was the complete opposite of my academic training. I instinctively began with and continue to use Scripture— specifically the drive and focus that is called for in Proverbs— as guidance and motivation for my research on the science of thought. This research produced my Switch On Your Brain 5-Step Learning Process (discussed in part 2), which teaches people to use disciplined, focused attention to develop the kind of thinking pattern that has huge benefits on attention networks and saves us from the enemy of distraction.

As a communication pathologist in the field of cognitive neuroscience, I saw the benefits of focused thinking and disciplined concentration were and are not just behavioral. Everything you do and say is first a thought in your physical brain.

You think, and then you do, which cycles back to the original thought, changing it and the thoughts connected to it in a dynamic interrelationship. If your thinking is off ("toxic" or "pathological," to be really sciency), then your communication through what you say and do is off, and vice versa. As the Scripture says, "As he thinks in his heart, so is he" (Prov. 23:7).

## Scientists See Evidence of the Difference

Scientists are seeing the evidence of deep, intellectual thought versus milkshake-multitasking in the brain.[8] Deep, intellectual thinking activates the prefrontal cortex (just above your eyebrows) in a positive way, producing increased concentration, less distraction, less switching between tasks, more effective switching between tasks, decreased emotional volatility, and overall increase in job completion.

Scientists have also found that deep, intellectual thinking improves connections within and between nerve networks, specifically in the front part of the brain and between the front and middle parts of the brain.[9] Other researchers found that when an individual pays attention to a stimulus, the neurons in the cerebral cortex that represent this object show increased attention.[10] We can also alter these patterns of activity by altering our attention, which remaps the cortex.

## Determination Is Key

During the 1990s, when many neuroscientists were reporting on the power of attention, I saw the greatest changes in patients who willfully, determinedly, and persistently chose to focus their attention on improving their skills and restoring function. For example, one of my patients had been in a car accident when she was a junior in high school that had left her with extreme brain damage. Her neurologist and other doctors told her parents not to raise their hopes of her being more than "a vegetable." Even when she got back to a fourth-grade level, the doctors said that was her limit. Fortunately she and her family chose not to pay attention to what they said and instead chose to focus her attention on what she wanted for her life. She was determined not only to correct her disabilities from the traumatic accident but also to catch up with her peer group and finish her senior year with them. Consequently, she built new networks in her mind focused on where she wanted to be and strove to make it happen.

She talked with me about her goals and vision, and we worked together, taking small steps, working consistently toward achieving them. There were times she wanted to give up, but she always picked herself up and carried on. The benefits were evident: Not only did she catch up with her peer group, but she also went on to complete twelfth grade and further her studies after high school. When we applied the various behavioral and neuropsychological tests after her period of therapy and compared them to her functioning before the accident, she had not only restored her original level but had gone way beyond in her functioning.[11]

What I believe happened to this patient is captured in two Scriptures: "Nothing they have imagined they could do would be impossible for them" (Gen. 11:6 AMP), and "Faith is the substance of things hoped for, the evidence of things not seen" (Heb. 11:1). To think positively about our prospects, we must be able to imagine ourselves in the future. Our brains may have stamps from the past, but they are being rewired by our expectation of the future. Imagining a positive future reduces the pain of the past. Faith motivates us to pursue these goals.

Hope leads to expectation, which creates peace, excitement, and health in our minds, thus increasing brain and body health.

## Additional Benefits of *Not* Milkshake-Multitasking

An additional benefit from deep thinking is increased *gyrification*, a lovely word that means more folds in the cortex of the brain. These extra folds allow the brain to process information faster, make decisions quicker, and improve memory.[12] Researchers specifically found an increase in folds in the insula, which is an amazing structure that integrates thinking, emotions, and self-regulation.[13] These studies show once again that the more you apply a pattern of deep, intellectual thought in your brain, the more you will improve the physical structure of your brain. Clearly, then, the parts of the brain involved in attention monitoring, working memory (dorsolateral prefrontal cortex), and how well we monitor our own thoughts (insula) and feelings improves dramatically with deep, intellectual thought.[14]

## Conclusion

These are just a few of the studies that show us that when we discipline our thoughts, positive, physical brain changes happen. This allows us to become more aligned with God's way of thinking: "Commit your works to the Lord, and your *thoughts* will be established" (Prov. 16:3, emphasis mine). Then we will switch between tasks correctly; monitor our attention, feelings, and thoughts; and function at a higher level. I just love that every instruction God gives us that we actually follow comes with a bonus physically and mentally. You do what God says and peace, happiness, and intelligence will follow.

## Chapter 6 Summary

1. The truth about multitasking is that it is a persistent myth.

2. What we really do is shift our attention rapidly and haphazardly from task to task, resulting in two negative things: (1) We don't devote as much focused attention as we should to a specific activity, task, or piece of information, and (2) we sacrifice the quality of our attention. I call this *milkshake-multitasking*.

3. This milkshake-multitasking creates patterns of flightiness and lack of concentration that unfortunately are often erroneously labeled ADD and ADHD. Too often this results in unnecessary medication, which adds fuel to the fire.

4. The general pattern today is that so much attention is paid to tweeting, Instagramming, and Facebooking that we forget all about enjoying the moment.

5. So-called social media experts tell us that information needs to be provided in bite-size amounts and in a constant stream of new information before the previous information has even been digested. This is not stimulation; it is bombardment.

6. Milkshake-multitasking decreases our attention, making us increasingly less able to focus on our thought habits. This opens us up to shallow and weak judgments and decisions, and it results in passive mindlessness.

7. Scientists are seeing the evidence of deep, intellectual thought versus milkshake-multitasking in the brain.

8. I saw the greatest changes in patients who willfully, determinedly, and persistently chose to focus their attention on improving their skills and restoring function.

# 7

# Thinking, God, and the Quantum Physics Brain

**Main Scripture:** Today I have given you the choice between life and death, between blessings and curses. Now I call on heaven and earth to witness the choice you make. Oh, that you would choose life, so that you and your descendants might live! Deuteronomy 30:19 NLT

**Linked Science Concepts:** The process of thinking and choosing is the most powerful thing in the universe after God, and it is a phenomenal gift from God to be treasured and used properly. The basic ingredients of quantum physics are: paying attention, thinking and choosing, and consequence.

As we have explored in previous chapters, our mind activity—the thoughts driven by the power of feelings—are the designers of the landscape of our brains. Thinking and choosing play a central role in who God has made us to be. In linking thought, choice, and science, quantum theory comes up as a star player.

The process of thinking and choosing is the most powerful thing in the universe after God, and it is a phenomenal gift from God to be treasured and used properly.

## Three Different Worlds

There is the sensory world of our five senses; there is the world of electromagnetism and the atom; and then there is the subatomic quantum world. This quantum world challenged physicists' perception of linear time, orderly space, and fixed realities and turned on its head the Cartesian Newtonian world that sees humans as machines with exchangeable parts.

This is God's style: Just when humans think they are super smart and know it all, a whole lot of new information enters into the equation and changes everything. In the words of Max Planck, the German theoretical physicist who won the Nobel Prize in 1918 for originating quantum theory, "Science progresses funeral by funeral."[1]

## Quantum Physics Is Another Way of Admiring God

*Quantum physics* is a way of explaining how the things that make up atoms work and makes sense of how the smallest things in nature work. *Quantum* means "energy," and quantum physics tells us how electromagnetic waves—like light waves—and particles work. *Quantum mechanics* is the mathematical framework used to describe this energy and how it works.

Using quantum physics, scientists can describe, predict, and quantify how we choose among a myriad of options. This is a way of *measuring* free will or describing it using a mathematical formula. In essence, quantum physics says that

- your consciousness affects the behaviors of subatomic particles;
- particles move backward and forward in time and appear in all possible places at once; and
- the universe is connected with transfers of information that are faster than light.

## Quantum Physics Aligning with Scripture

Quantum theory converts science's conception of humans from being mere cogs in a gigantic, mechanical machine to being freethinking agents whose conscious choices affect the physical world.[2] This is called the *observer effect*: The observer determines the direction in which the possibilities may collapse. In the quantum universe, as we—the observers—affect phenomena, space, and time, we turn possibilities into realities. Mind changes matter.

Here is a simple way of understanding this observer effect. Each day as you go through the events and circumstances of life, you are faced with a multitude of possibilities to choose, from what to wear in the morning to how you are going to react to the email you have just received. There is an endless array of possible choices you can make at any one moment in time, but it is you, with your ability to think, who directs the choice. So you collapse all the probabilities into one choice: "eggs for breakfast," "I will not be upset by the tone of this email," or "I will not say *can't* today." So as you choose, you collapse the probability into an actuality. Satan, the father of lies (John 8:44), will come at you with a thousand negative probabilities, but you always need to remember that a probability has no power. It only becomes powerful when you believe the lie and collapse the probability into an actuality. This is how evil is birthed.

## Free Will—A Basic Ingredient of Quantum Physics

Quantum physics has as its basic ingredients free will, directed attention as the result of a choice, and the effects and consequences of these choices. For example, Proverbs 4:20–27 says that if we direct our attention to the Word of God, we will align our thinking and subsequent choices with God, and the outcome will be healing and health.

Thus an intentional act—such as choosing to attend to God's words, listen to them, memorize them—will produce the effect of health to all your flesh. Deuteronomy 30:19 (NIV) can be evaluated in the same way: "I have set before you life and death, blessings and curses"—the options—"Now choose life"—you intentionally evaluate the options and choose your reaction—"so that you and your children may live"—which is the consequence of your intentional choice.

Let's apply the basic ingredients of quantum physics: paying attention, thinking and choosing, and consequence.

1. Information: You get a call from your doctor's office telling you that the results of your blood test are in and asking you to phone them as soon as possible.
2. Thoughts: Multiple thoughts are swirling around in your head. Option one is fear: "They said as soon as possible! Does this mean bad news? What if I have . . ."

And on it goes, down to planning the songs for your funeral. Option two is denial: "This is routine; I'll call when I have time." Option three is trust: "I have faith that this will be good news. I am not moved by any doctor's report."

3. Choice: You choose an option. For instance, if you choose fear, your brain responds by wiring in the thought, "I am sick," and you live into this thought.

4. Consequence: You suddenly feel sick and are sure you are dying.

5. New consequence: You phone the doctor; your results are clear; and suddenly you feel fine (and perhaps a little foolish).

So your brain becomes what you focused on (body carries out the will of the spirit and soul), and what your brain has become produces what you say and do and how you feel physically and mentally.[3]

## The Granddaddy of Definitions

Quantum physics has multiple definitions, but the original Copenhagen formulation of quantum theory made by Niehls Bohr of Copenhagen University in 1927 is considered the *granddaddy* of the definitions.[4] It states that the free choices made by human subjects are a subjectively controllable variable, which simply means that you control your choices. Quantum mechanics can be used to prove that thinking and choosing are real and measurable.[5] The way you experience your feelings, the way you interface with your thoughts, and the kind of attention you give them will change how your brain functions.

If you apply this principle, you can free yourself from destructive thoughts and actions and change bad habits for good.

## The Quantum Zeno Effect

I love quantum physics, but the quantum physics principle that really caught my attention is called the Quantum Zeno Effect (QZE). QZE is the repeated effort that causes learning to take place. When you go over and over something, reading it, thinking about it, writing it down, and then repeating this process, you deepen your knowledge and understanding, direct your attention, and grow nerve cells. The neurons in your brain line up and fire together because you are firing synapses over and over, which causes genetic expression to happen and makes the synapses and proteins stronger. The changes in your brain caused by this deep, repeated, intellectually targeted focus can be seen with brain imaging techniques.[6]

Basically, the QZE stipulates that your brain becomes *what* you focus on and *how* you focus. So the consequence is structural change in the brain that produces behavior because we operate from what we have built into our brain. Choosing to pay selective attention to and focus on what you are gathering in through your five senses acts on the physical structure of the brain, amplifying activity in particular brain circuits.

In my research and clinical practice I have trained teachers and students how to direct their attention in a systematic, organized, logical way that followed how the brain builds thought. This incorporated gathering the relevant information, reading it over and over, thinking about it over and over, writing it down, checking through it all again for accuracy, teaching it out loud, and applying it. I call this my 5-Step Switch On Your Brain Learning Process. In my PhD research, my control group was the historical academic trend of the school, which used basic study skills intervention and a traditional teaching and learning approach. Once I introduced my Switch On Your Brain Process to a group of students, their academic trend significantly improved. The results showed a 35 to 70 percent improvement in metacognitive and cognitive performance as measured by academic results in four subjects: English, math, history, and science.[7] These students had developed the attitude that persistence and hard work would achieve an end result, and that stretching themselves and challenging their minds is what would make the change. They learned the science behind this in their sessions with me and applied the lessons in their academics—and the results spoke for themselves. This was essentially the Quantum Zeno Effect in action, which I have also seen repeatedly in my other research, the lives of my patients, my children, and even my own life. I have successfully worked with clients as young as three and as old as seventy-eight—a pilot who wanted to change professions and become a CPA.

Part of what I taught these students in their first session was an understanding that intelligence is continually developing, so they could become as intelligent as they wanted to be, based on how much they used their brains. Part of this session also included a basic introduction into how the brain works when we learn and how to build memory, including the concept of neuroplasticity. An important fact I explained was that they were *in control* of the development of their own brains, and that hard work and challenging themselves helped the brain grow more brain cells. Their motivation and enthusiasm for taking responsibility for their own learning was incredible.

Dr. Carol Dweck, a Stanford University research psychologist, found similar results. She found that students who believed that intelligence can grow had increasing math scores. Those that believed that intelligence was fixed experienced a decrease in their math scores. She then compared a group of students who were trained in basic study skills to another group who were told how their brains grow in response to novelty and challenge. At the end of the semester, those who had the "mini neuroscience" approach had significantly better math grades than the other group.[8]

## The Law of Entanglement

The *law of entanglement* in quantum physics states that relationship is the defining characteristic of everything in space and time. Because of the pervasive nature of the entanglement of atomic particles, the relationship is independent of distance and requires no physical link. Everything and everyone is linked, and we all affect each other.

The law of entanglement has a biblical correlation: "So we, being many, are one body in Christ, and individually members one of another" (Rom. 12:5). If you are not doing what God put you on this earth to do—your divine sense of purpose (Eccles. 3:11)—then even though you may not know me, you are still affecting my life. We are all part of God, so this interconnectedness is not surprising. Your intentions, your prayers, and your words toward others will have impact because of this law. We see this in the Scriptures: "The effectual fervent prayer of a righteous man availeth much" (James 5:16 KJV). In fact, we are so entangled that our intentions alter not only our own DNA molecules, but the DNA molecules of others as well. An ingenuous experiment set up by the HeartMath Foundation determined that genuine positive emotion, as reflected by a measure called "heart rate variability," directed with intentionality toward someone actually changed the way the double-helix DNA strand coils and uncoils. And this goes for both positive and negative emotions and intentions.[9] Other research shows that even thirty seconds a day of direct heartfelt intention will cumulatively alter not only your own destiny, but impact the lives of others in this generation and the next three at least.[10]

Look at the story of the woman in Matthew 9:20–22 who bled for twelve years. She was so desperate for her healing that when she heard about the man called Jesus who heals, she started directing her intentions with each bit of information she received, cumulatively building a physical thought in her mind of her healing and believing it in her heart—in effect she was applying Genesis 11:6 and Hebrews 11:1. In this way she developed her faith and aligned herself with the healing power of God, and in doing so she built a root thought (Proverbs 23:7) and acted upon it to receive her healing. She collapsed all the probabilities into one, which said, "I will be healed if I just touch the hem of his garment." Furthermore, her entanglement with God (Colossians 1:16) was activated by her choice to believe in her heart and confess with her mouth. There was no cognitive dissonance in her that day, meaning she wasn't thinking one thing and confessing another. Science shows the beauty of what happens when we align with God. Science is a way God shows us that we are part of him, and when we follow his laws we reap the benefit.

I honestly believe that by applying our intelligence, which can be developed and trained, we can become amazingly good at understanding how to practice the presence of God. I have personally reached a point where science has taken my relationship with God to a whole new level. He has become very real and very personal. Through science, you see how much trouble he has gone to in order to show himself to us in every way possible.

We are entangled in each other's lives, and this is reflected in the structure of the brain. We have "mirror neurons" that fire up as we watch someone else laugh or cry or drink a cup of coffee. Giacomo Rizzolatti and his team were the first to discover these mirror neurons in 1995.[11] Through these neurons we literally fire up activity in the brain without actually using our five senses through the normal sensory-cognitive cycle. Empathy is the wonderful God-given ability to identify with, and vicariously understand, the internal experiences of another person, making communication more genuine and valuable.[12] When we empathize, many different regions of the brain collaborate in addition to the tiny, miraculous mirror neurons. We have been hardwired to experience powerful compassion for others, and this compassion crosses all three worlds: sensory, electromagnetic, and quantum.

## Particles Behave in a Bizarre Way, Which Is Another Reason Why Prayer Works

Quantum theory calls entanglement "bizarre behavior" for particles—such as two entangled particles behaving as one even when far apart. Physicists call such behavior *nonlocal*, which means that it is physically impossible to know the position and the momentum of a particle at the same time. Another way of saying this is that there is no space-time dimension.

We know God operates outside of the space-time dimension. And we know prayer does too. There are many stories of people praying for each other on different sides of the planet and experiencing the effect of the prayer. In fact, there are many documented studies on the impact of prayer in the world of neuroscience in addition to the millions of testimonies from Christians around the world.

An innovative experiment was done that showed that we are capable of impacting each other's minds and brains even when sensory signals (the five senses), electromagnetic signals, mirror neurons, and insula activity have all been removed. This impact only worked with meditators who had built a relationship with each other, not those in the control group who didn't have a relationship. In the experiment researchers got two people to meditate next to each other in an electronically shielded room, called a "faraday cage." Then they separated them into two separate faraday cages, and as they continued to meditate, researchers shone light in the eye of one of the meditators. The part of the brain that lit up in that person's brain also lit up in the other meditator's brain, even though there was no sensory or electromagnetic connection.[13]

Classical physics says this could only work if there were a prior arrangement—something like, "If this happens, then that will happen." So no space-time dimension seems to violate our sense of cause and effect in space and time. For example, if someone needs heart surgery, then heart surgery is performed and is either successful or not. However, one study showed that those undergoing heart surgery who had spiritual support in the form of prayer and social support showed a mortality rate one seventh of those who did not.[14] Other researchers found that those who attended church regularly and had a stronger faith were less likely to die and had better overall health.[15] There are over *twelve hundred* studies linking intentional prayer and overall health and longevity.[16] Meta-analyses in various medical journals have compiled results that show that intentional prayer significantly affects healing.[17] Dr. David Levy, a practicing neurosurgeon in California, prays for his patients before he operates on them and has amazing results. The majority of his patients want him to pray because it shows them he cares more about their health and about them as a person than a physician who does not discuss spiritual matters with his or her patients.[18]

I love what Dr. Levy says about how he approaches the often life-threatening and frightening brain surgeries that his patients face:

> I have been in this profession for a good number of years and am intimately familiar with most of the new therapies, medical devices, and drugs hitting the market. Many of them are ingenious, and I use them regularly in my practice. I have consulted for several companies to develop better devices and have travelled the world teaching others to use them. I admire and am grateful for modern medical technology. But though technology can prolong a life or reduce pain, it cannot always make life better. My experiences have convinced me that spirituality is a crucial element to the wellbeing of a person as a whole; moreover if we let him, God can do powerful, supernatural things in our everyday lives. That's why I began inviting God into my consultations, exams and surgeries. Many would be surprised that a neurosurgeon—a man of science, logic and human progress—would be such a strong believer in God and divine intervention. Yet the experience has been nothing short of phenomenal.[19]

This experiment highlights how we impact each other through our intentions and prayers. Our prayers impact each other, but so do the negative words we speak over people we are in relationship with. However, we need to remember that "a curse without cause shall not alight" (Prov. 26:2).

## Matter Just Keeps Getting Smaller

We have gone from molecules to atoms to quarks, leptons, and bosons; and now physicists are proposing an even smaller concept called *preons* as minuscule particles that make up quarks. They are also proposing a string theory, which says that the ultimate building blocks of matter are tiny, vibrating strings, which are even smaller than preons. One scientist even describes preons as twisted braids of space-time.[20] If preons exist (I think they do), they are unimaginably tiny and would have to fit inside a quark, which is currently the smallest known particle of matter, having a size of zero, and the strings are even smaller.[21]

## Thought Moves Faster Than the Speed of Light

Electrons have been observed to jump from one orbit to another without traveling through the intervening space and without time having elapsed.

Scientists say our thought signals also seem to move faster than the speed of light and in ways that classical physics cannot explain. How else do you explain the effect we have on each other, how someone with a negative attitude impacts how you feel?

Remember the mirror neurons in the brain that mirror each other's emotions, facilitating empathy that I spoke about a few paragraphs back? These signals that are passed between us are made up of energy that can be explained—at this time, anyway—in terms of quantum physics.

## A Glimpse into the Spiritual World

These observations also give us a glimpse of the spiritual side of the world that is beyond time and space. It could explain how, after Jesus's resurrection, he appeared to two men on the road to Emmaus, then later that evening as soon as they recognized who he was, he suddenly disappeared (Luke 24:31).

A few verses further on in Luke's Gospel, Jesus suddenly appeared among the disciples, and they thought he was a ghost (Luke 24:36–46). Later, Philip suddenly disappears after the Ethiopian's baptism (Acts 8:28–40). These are all mysteries that quantum physics hints at solving, as though God is reeling us in with beautiful and fascinating concepts to try to explain these mysteries.

## Unpredictability Is the Norm

Unpredictability is the norm and therefore requires faith and "without faith it is impossible to please God" (Heb. 11:6 NIV). We see this concept in the *Heisenberg uncertainty principle*, which is a radical departure from classical physics in that it replaces dogmatic certainty with ambiguity.

For example, humans are seen as observers outside the system[22] who exert an effect that is unpredictable. And it is not just humans who are unpredictable. The unpredictability reaches down to the level of electrons and photons of light, which cannot have a definite momentum or position at the same time; particles are neither particles nor waves because they are both. And as for quarks, bosons, and now preons and strings, they are simply all over the place.

## Quantum Physics Math Predictions
## Show Unpredictability

You can try to mathematically predict uncertainty. (Sounds strange, doesn't it?) Quantum physics math prediction is all about mathematically showing this uncertainty, which basically undergirds free will.[23] But you will never be 100 percent accurate in predicting exactly what another person is thinking—even someone you know very well.

This is a God-ordained precept in which it is clear that no human knows another human's thoughts except that person and God. "For what man knows the things of a man except the spirit of the man which is in him? Even so no one knows the things of God except the Spirit of God" (1 Cor. 2:11).

The weather tomorrow, what your friend is going to say, what you will be doing at this time a week from today, in fact all aspects of life in the future—these all follow Heisenberg's uncertainty principle. It gives us two options: faith or fear. I don't know what you are going to choose, but obviously I hope it will be faith. Why worry about tomorrow? Your heavenly Father knows what you need (Matt. 6:25–33).

## It's All about Trusting That God Is Who He Says He Is

Heisenberg's uncertainty principle is a nightmare for classical physicists and others who try to explain away God and free will. Einstein, who could never reconcile himself to this random aspect of nature, famously pronounced, "*Der Alte wurfelt nicht,*" which is translated, "The old man, that is God, does not play dice." Well, God is not playing dice; he is simply telling us to trust him and stop trying to control everything, which is a full-blown setback for the notion that the future can be accurately forecast. One cannot fathom the intent of God (Ps. 145:3; Eccles. 3:1; Rom. 11:33).

Einstein simply looked at it from the wrong angle. The correct angle is found in Scripture: "Trust in the LORD with all your heart and lean not on your own understanding. In all your ways acknowledge Him, and he will direct your paths" (Prov. 3:5–6), and "Many are the plans in the mind of a man, but it is the purpose of the LORD that will stand" (Prov. 19:21 ESV).

American physicist Don Lincoln, a ground-breaking researcher of particle physics at Fermi National Accelerator Laboratory, captures very succinctly and clearly what I believe God is doing in science:

> We can move easily through air but not through a wall. The sun transmutes one element to another, bathing our planet in warmth and light. Radio waves have carried man's voice to earth from the surface of the moon, whereas gamma rays can inflict fatal damage on our DNA. On the face of it, these disparate phenomena have nothing to do with one another, but physicists have uncovered a handful of principles that fuse into a theory of sublime simplicity to explain all this and much more. This theory is called the standard model of particle physics, and it encapsulates the electromagnetic forces that make a wall feel solid, the nuclear forces that govern the sun's power plant, and the diverse family of light waves that both make modern communications possible and threaten our well-being.[24]

## God's Plans

Quantum physics, and neuroscience for that matter, do not provide ultimate answers; they are simply stepping-stones in the development of our understanding of our Almighty God, another way of admiring God. Just as sound waves across the air or big metal planes flying in the sky or nuclear power were inconceivable before the discovery of atomic structure, so would unveiling a new layer of matter or a new, complex brain circuit or a biochemical pathway or a better understanding of genes reveal phenomena we cannot even begin to imagine. God pulls us along in exciting suspense in this enjoyable discovery of his creation. He is trying to show us that "glory belongs to God, whose power is at work in us. By this power he can do infinitely more than we can ask or imagine" (Eph. 3:20 GW).

Let me point out the obvious: God created everything, and that includes science and physics, and he has revealed the laws of this material world we live in over the ages to help us understand him. I am not being a materialist; far from it. I believe God is taking us through the material world into the spiritual world to get to know him more deeply. Why, after all, did he put our soul and spirit in a physical body and place us in a physical world?

Quantum physics is creeping into every field, causing confusion among scientists, dealing a deathblow to the Newtonian dream, all because it points directly back to God, "the old man," who has ultimate control. I love it when his plans come together.

## Chapter 7 Summary

1. There is the sensory world of our five senses; there is the world of electromagnetism and the atom; and then there is the deeper quantum world.
2. This quantum world challenges physicists' perception of linear time, orderly space, and fixed realities; and it

turns on its head the Cartesian Newtonian world that sees humans as machines with exchangeable parts.

3. Quantum physics, which is different from classical physics, is a way of explaining how the things that make up atoms work and making sense of how the smallest things in nature work.

4. Quantum means *energy*, so quantum physics also tells us how electromagnetic waves—like light waves—work.

5. Quantum mechanics is the mathematical framework used to describe this energy and how it works.

6. Quantum physics basically says
   - your consciousness affects the behaviors of subatomic particles;
   - particles move backward and forward in time and appear in all possible places at once; and
   - the universe is connected with faster-than-light transfers of information.

7. Five main ideas are presented in quantum theory:
   - Energy is not a continuous stream but comes in small, discrete units.
   - The basic units behave both like particles and like waves.
   - The movement of these particles is random.
   - It is physically impossible to know both the position and the momentum of a particle at the same time.
   - The atomic world is nothing like the world we live in.

8. Quantum theory converts science's conception of humans from being mere cogs in a gigantic, mechanical machine to being freethinking agents whose conscious,

free choices affect the physical world. This is called the *observer effect*.

9. The Copenhagen interpretation of quantum theory says that the particle is what you measure it to be. This means our perceptions determine the outcome; we perceive the world through the thoughts (memories) we have built into our brains.

10. The Quantum Zeno Effect (QZE) is the repeated effort that causes learning to take place.

11. The *law of entanglement* in quantum physics states that relationship is the defining characteristic of everything in space and time. Because of the pervasive nature of the entanglement of atomic particles, relationship is independent of distance and requires no physical link. Everything and everyone is linked, and we all affect each other.

12. Thought signals seem to move faster than the speed of light and in ways that classical physics cannot explain. This means our mind controls matter and is therefore a creative force.

13. Humans are seen as observers outside the system who exert an effect that is *unpredictable*. And it is not just humans who are unpredictable. The unpredictability reaches down to the level of electrons and photons of light, which cannot have a definite momentum or position at the same time; particles are neither particles nor waves because they are both. And as for quarks, bosons, and now preons and strings—they are simply all over the place.

14. The random and unpredictable nature of quantum physics is called the *Heisenberg uncertainty principle*.

This principle is a way God shows us that we do not control the future. He does.

15. Quantum physics math prediction is all about mathematically showing this uncertainty, which basically undergirds free will.

16. I believe God is taking us through the material world into the spiritual world to get to know him more deeply, and the quantum concept is part of this journey.

# 8

# The Science of Thought

Main Scripture: Therefore put away all filthiness and rampant wickedness and receive with meekness the implanted word, which is able to save your souls. James 1:21 ESV

Linked Science Concept: What you wire into your brain through thinking is stored in your nonconscious mind. The nonconscious mind is where 99.9 percent of our mind activity is. It is the root level that stores the thoughts with the emotions and perceptions, and it impacts the conscious mind and what we say and do. Everything is first a thought. The Geodesic Information Processing Theory is a scientific way of understanding this.

The brain is not an input-output machine. You are not an input-output machine. You are not a computer mirroring the outside world. Your brain is designed to respond to your mind. You are intrinsically and brilliantly designed in the sense that your brain carries out the will of the spirit and the soul. Internal activity in your mind is where everything begins, "for as he thinks in his heart, so is he" (Prov. 23:7).

## The Power of Your Thought Life

In my research, I spent many years trying to understand science in terms of the truths of Scripture. I researched, developed, and tested a theory that can basically be described as explaining the science of thought—or in simple terms, how we think and the effect of our thoughts on our brain, body, and mind. I applied this in many ways with my patients and in my research over time.[1]

If you look at the image of my theory, "The Geodesic Information Processing Theory" on pages 126–27, it will help you understand this internal activity, the science of thought, a little better.

Before I explain this in a simple way, let me tell you why I am doing this. When you understand the power of your thought life, which has been the emphasis of the first seven chapters in this book, you truly begin to get a glimpse of how important it is to take responsibility for what you are thinking. Thinking is a powerful creative force, both a blessing and a curse, and should not be taken lightly. So, in exposing you to a tested scientific theory, albeit briefly in this chapter, I am giving you some tangible proof (not the only proof) that God was so serious about us capturing our thoughts and renewing our minds that he gave us science as encouragement.

Thomas More explains this so well in his book *Utopia*:

> The scientific investigation of nature is not only a most enjoyable process but also the best possible means of pleasing the Creator. . . . He has the normal reactions of an artist.

Having put the marvelous system of the universe on show for human beings to look at—since no other species is capable of taking it in—He must prefer the type of person who examines it carefully, and really admires his work, to the type that just ignores it and like the lower animals remains quite unimpressed by the whole astonishing spectacle.[2]

You will see there are three levels on the schematic of my theory: (1) Nonconscious metacognitive level; (2) Conscious cognitive level; and (3) Symbolic output level.

### Nonconscious Metacognitive Level

The nonconscious metacognitive level is on the far left. It is where 90 to 99 percent of the action in your mind is; your thinking and thought-building happen on this level. This level operates at about four hundred billion actions per second and drives the conscious cognitive level. It operates twenty-four hours a day.

### Conscious Cognitive Level

The conscious cognitive level, in the middle, is where up to 10 percent of mind action is. It operates at about two thousand actions per second, so it is much slower and is controlled by the metacognitive level. The cognitive level in turn drives the symbolic output level (end section), which is what you say and do—what the world sees, the output of your thinking. This level operates when we are awake.

### Symbolic Action Level

The symbolic output level incorporates the five senses through which you express yourself and experience the world,

# THE GEODESIC INFORMATION PROCESSING MODEL

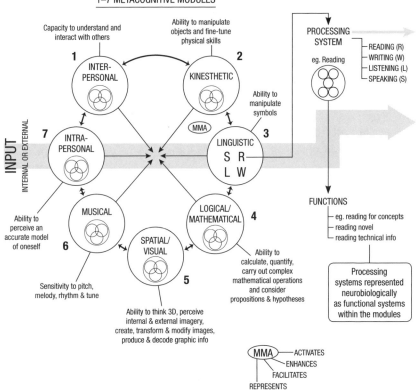

NON-CONSCIOUS

## METACOGNITIVE LEVEL

90% of Learning

MMA

Root of thinking process and then structure of the non-conscious → Automatized complex higher cortical functions

1–7 METACOGNITIVE MODULES

Capacity to understand and interact with others

**1**
INTER-PERSONAL

Ability to manipulate objects and fine-tune physical skills

**2**
KINESTHETIC

Ability to manipulate symbols

MMA

**3**
LINGUISTIC
S R
L W

PROCESSING SYSTEM
eg. Reading
— READING (R)
— WRITING (W)
— LISTENING (L)
— SPEAKING (S)

INPUT
INTERNAL OR EXTERNAL

**7**
INTRA-PERSONAL

Ability to perceive an accurate model of oneself

**6**
MUSICAL

Sensitivity to pitch, melody, rhythm & tune

SPATIAL/VISUAL
**5**

Ability to think 3D, perceive internal & external imagery, create, transform & modify images, produce & decode graphic info

LOGICAL/MATHEMATICAL **4**

Ability to calculate, quantify, carry out complex mathematical operations and consider propositions & hypotheses

FUNCTIONS
— eg. reading for concepts
— reading novel
— reading technical info

Processing systems represented neurobiologically as functional systems within the modules

MMA —ACTIVATES
—ENHANCES
—FACILITATES
REPRESENTS

## NEUROPSYCHOLOGICAL LEVEL

BIOLOGICAL REPRESENTATION

1–7 represented biologically as modular colums of neuronal cells ascending from the cortex to the subcortex to the limbic system across the left and right hemispheres

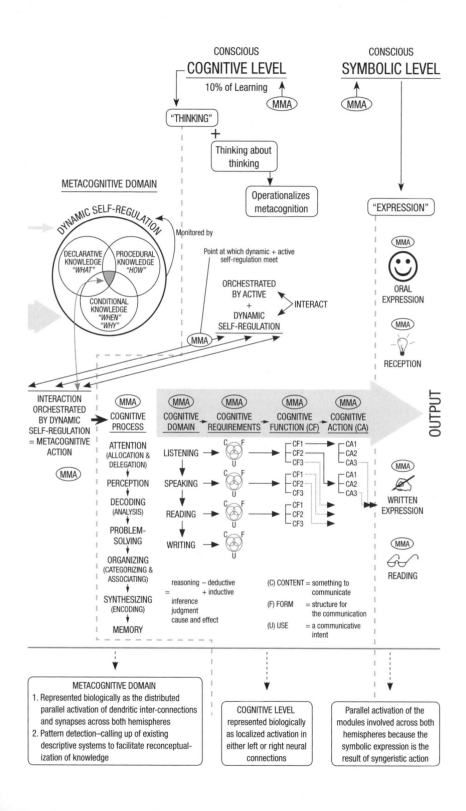

serving as the contact between the external world and the internal world of your mind. Therefore, this model works in reverse as well, forming a perfect circle. So information comes through the five senses, is received consciously by the conscious cognitive level, and then passes into the nonconscious meta-cognitive level where—if you have paid attention and started thinking and choosing—it becomes a physical thought as a result of genetic expression (the making of proteins). This newly built physical thought will, in turn, impact your conscious cognitive and symbolic levels—and so the cycle goes on.

## 21-Day Brain Detox Plan

Whatever you think about the most will grow, so the more the cycle moves with a particular thought, the stronger it grows. This is in essence the Quantum Zeno Effect (QZE) taking place that I explained in chapter 7. It takes around twenty-one days of this cycling for all the necessary protein changes[3] to happen to create a long-term integrated memory.

This is why my brain detox plan is for twenty-one days. You can't just apply a thought once and think change has happened. It takes repeated work for the QZE to take effect. Each day something is happening to the thought in your non-conscious mind. So if you stop at day 4 or 5, which is often when people do give up, then the consequence will be that the memory denatures—which means it dies and becomes heat energy. Simply put, you forget.

## You Feel the Pull

It's important to note that we feel the pull of the sensory information coming in through the symbolic level, but we don't have to go there. These are the events and circumstances from the outside world. The events and circumstances from the outside world also enter into our minds and brains through electromagnetic and the quantum worlds (chap. 7). Remember, we cannot control the events and circumstances of our lives, but we *can control our reactions*. Don't be reactive; take time to slow down and think (see chaps. 4, 5, and 6).

Our five senses activate an emotional response almost immediately, but if we don't take the time to process them, the unprocessed emotion will dominate. This is why all the keys I am describing in part 1 of this book are so important; they help you deal with this pull.

Satan tries to take advantage of the pull of the five senses through this symbolic level, and he would love it if you respond impulsively to them. But you are made in God's image with the mind of Christ, and Jesus told his disciples that all power had been given to him (Matt. 28:18). If all power was given to Jesus, how much power does Satan have? None. When you truly let that sink in, you will realize that you control your reactions, your thinking, and your choices.

## What Lies Are You Believing?

It's through the senses that we receive Satan's lies, but—and this is important—we don't have to believe those lies. If we do believe them, we process them into physical realities (through the conscious cognitive to the nonconscious metacognitive) that form the substance of the nerve networks upon which we act. This means that if we listen to and believe the Enemy's lies, we actually choose to process them into physical realities inside our brains. In doing so, we create the evil and act upon it. But we do not have to believe Satan's lies. We as humans create evil when we collapse these probabilities into actualities (chap. 7). So evil does not come from God, obviously, yet people often say that if God created everything, then he created evil as well. God has given us the power to create: this creative force can become good or evil through our choices.

Current neuroscientific and quantum physics research confirms that our thoughts change our brains daily. In fact, neurological literature has coined the term "self-directed neuroplasticity" as a general description of the principle that deep thinking changes brain structure and function.[4] This plastic ability of the brain to change in a positive or negative direction depending on our state of mind is called the *plastic paradox*. Positive plasticity produces positive behavior, and negative plasticity produces negative behaviors.

## Distorted Love and Truth Get Wired In

When we distort love and truth, we wire this perversion into our brains and, in a sense, create brain damage. This is not an exaggeration, because our brains are wired for love, not fear, and therefore all the circuits—neurochemical, neurophysiological, neurobiological, electromagnetic, and quantum—are geared up for healthy, not toxic, thinking. If we allow ourselves to learn fear, it creates chaos and havoc in our brains.[5]

For example, one study showed that when patients with OCD remained toxic, obsessing and worrying about an issue, their brains showed damage and incorrect firing.[6] The researcher saw a decrease in activity in the lateral prefrontal cortex (just above your temples) where the circuits would normally have generated and maintained strategy. The medial orbital frontal cortex (behind your eyes) became more imbalanced and busy, which meant their decision-making ability became impaired. In addition, the amygdala (deep inside the middle of your brain running backward from the corner of your eyes) showed less balanced activity, so the patients were not evaluating emotional significance correctly. All this negative brain activity changed positively once the researcher put the patients through a rigid, directed, mental activity program.

If you look back to the chart of my theory again (see pp. 126–27), the bottom part beneath the horizontal line represents the neurological level that I have been describing throughout this book. Essentially the first three levels all describe mind activity, and the bottom level shows that this mind activity signals a change in brain structure. So my theory, the Geodesic Information Processing Theory, falls within the realm of cognitive neuroscience.

I show in my theory that the brain works in neurological pillars and multiple parallel circuits, which means there is a lot of interconnectivity among the neurons.[7] Essentially, the Geodesic Information Processing Theory deals with the science of thought. It is a description of how we think, choose, and build thoughts and the impact of this on our brain and behavior. It is our choices that make something out of nothing. This is basically cognitive neuroscience in action: the mind-brain connection.

My Switch On Your Brain 21-Day Brain Detox Plan, which is based on my theory and research, is designed to help improve your thinking and choices and subsequent happiness and health. It is our choices that create healthy thought universes in our brain, or they turn the powerless lie into a toxic thought universe in our brain. This is the incredible power God has given us: to be able to think and choose and create reality.

### Automatization and Riding a Bicycle

After a period of repeated thinking about a choice over two to three cycles of twenty-one days, the new thought moves into the nonconscious metacognitive level, where it becomes part of our internal perception. This process is called *automatization*.

A simple example of automatization is learning to ride a bike. Initially, it was difficult and you wobbled all around. But as you practiced with determination—which means you applied the QZE—and intensely concentrated on the sequence of how to ride a bike, suddenly one day you were riding perfectly. It appeared as though having mastered the skill of bike riding meant you were not thinking about the process of cycling because now you rode the bike automatically. But you were actually thinking very nonconsciously—I know that makes no sense yet, so read on.

All the focused, dedicated, and repeated practice you consciously put into the learning process over time created a very strong thought network. Once the skill was mastered with the repeated and focused practice, it moved from the conscious mind (cognitive level) to the nonconscious mind (metacognitive level). Even though you were not consciously aware of the how-to-ride-a-bicycle thought, it was very much alive, and it was the guiding force behind the cycling. So each time you got on your bike, this memory was still in your metacognitive nonconscious guiding your bicycle riding. And as you ride around on your bike, you bring that thought into your conscious mind and it becomes malleable (plastic and changeable), and a few new branches are added as you cycle over that challenging mountain path or speed-jump over a log trying to keep up with your teenage son. So when you get off that bike, that "cycling thought" has become enriched from the experience you have just gone through.

## Automatization Is a Life Principle

Automatization applies to everything in your life, because everything you do and say is first a thought. This means *nothing happens* until you first build the thought, which is like the root of a tree buried under the ground. The thought produces words, actions, behavior, and so on, which can be compared to the tree, branches, leaves, flowers, and fruit you see above the ground. The roots under the ground are like the nonconscious metacognitive mind that nourishes and supports the tree, keeping it alive twenty-four hours a day.[8] The nonconscious metacognitive mind operates and nourishes your conscious cognitive mind twenty-four hours a day.

The nonconscious metacognitive mind is filled with the thoughts you have been building since you were in the womb, and they form the perceptual base from which you see life. Up to 99 percent of the decisions you make are based on what you have built and automatized into your nonconscious metacognitive level.[9] If a person's nonconscious metacognitive mind is filled with negative, toxic trash, then that is what informs his or her decisions on a day-to-day basis, which means that person will speak and act from toxicity. This is metacognitive to cognitive to symbolic—as per my theory.

Obviously the opposite of toxicity is health, and we were originally designed by God for health because we are made in God's image (Gen. 1:26). So we begin with health and then move away through bad choices. Most of the time we are a mix of healthy and toxic—you determine the proportions of these two for yourself.

You cannot sit back and wait to be happy and healthy and have a great thought life; you have to make the choice to make this happen. You have to choose to get rid of the toxic and get back in alignment with God. You can be overwhelmed by every small setback in life, or you can be energized by the possibilities they bring.

## Chapter 8 Summary

1. The Geodesic Information Processing Theory deals with the science of thought. It is a description of how we think, choose, and build thoughts and the impact of this on our brain and behavior.

2. I show in my Geodesic Information Processing Theory that the brain works in neurological pillars and multiple parallel circuits, which means there is a lot of interconnectivity among the networks of the brain.

3. It is our choices that make something out of nothing. It's our choices that collapse the probabilities into actualities that define the state of our nonconscious metacognition, which in turn inform our conscious cognition and symbolic actions.

4. My Switch On Your Brain 21-Day Brain Detox Plan, which is based on my theory and research, is designed to help improve your thinking and choices and subsequent happiness and health.

5. It is our choices that either create healthy thought universes in our brain or turn the powerless lie into a toxic thought universe—which is essentially evil. This is the incredible power God has given us: to be able to think and choose and create reality. This reality can be good or evil based on our choices.

6. After a period of repeated thinking about the choice over two to three cycles of twenty-one days, the new thought moves into the nonconscious metacognitive

level where it becomes part of our internal perception. This process is called *automatization*.

7. Everything you do and say is first a thought.
8. The nonconscious metacognitive mind is filled with the thoughts you have been building since you were born, and they form the perceptual base from which you see life.

Now, as you move into part 2 of this book, remember the eight keys from chapters 1 through 8 and refer back to them often to get the most out of the 21-Day Brain Detox:

1. Mind controls matter
2. Choice and your multiple-perspective advantage
3. Your choices change your brain
4. Catch those thoughts
5. Entering into directed rest
6. Stop milkshake-multitasking
7. Thinking, God, and the quantum physics brain
8. The science of thought

Now step into part 2 and switch on your brain!

# The 21-Day Brain Detox Plan

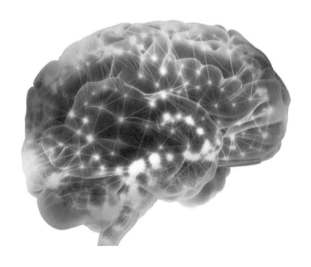

# 9

# What Is the 21-Day
# Brain Detox Plan?

The hardest part about achieving peak happiness, thinking, and health is remembering that we can choose them. Achieving them is not accomplished by putting on a brave or happy face, nor are they attained by adopting an ostrich mentality and pretending that problems don't exist or that everything will always be great. The way to find this state is by harnessing the neuroplasticity God has designed in our brains and choosing to rewire—or renew—our mind (Rom. 12:2). This is a lifestyle that will bring us ever closer in alignment to our original design of perfection (Matt. 5:48), of being made in God's image (Gen. 1:26).

We can actively choose happiness rather than letting our external and internal world of wired-in and learned thoughts and our biology define happiness for us. We need to wire in positive thought networks that can fill us with the power to get us back on track (2 Tim. 1:7). It is the implanted Word that will save our souls (James 1:21). Who we are is where happiness lies, but this is so often blocked by who we have become.

## A Simple Tool That Brings Peace

Even though the 21-Day Brain Detox Plan is based on rigorous science and the Word of God, it is a simple tool to help bring peak happiness, thinking, health, and peace—not only into your life but also into the lives of your loved ones. To detox your thought life, you need to remember *it's your thinking that will actually change your brain*. So you need to do *consciously* what your brain does on a *nonconscious* level to build a thought. You control your brain; your brain does not control you.

## A Simple Brain Sequence That Makes Things Happen

In order to make this nonconscious to conscious process happen effectively, what you do each day is my 5-Step Switch On Your Brain Learning Process. This is a "brain sequence" based on my Geodesic Information Processing Theory, which describes the science of thought (see chap. 8). This is a statistically significant and scientifically proven technique that I developed many years ago and have continued to develop and use over the years in my research and clinical experience to help people think and learn for lasting success. It is based on complex science that focuses on the dynamics of the thought process. In this book I will teach you the simple application, but more thorough details can be found in my scientific references if you wish to read further.[1]

## The 5-Step Switch On Your Brain Learning Process

The 5-Step Switch On Your Brain Learning Process has at its heart focused, organized, and disciplined deep intellectual thinking to break down toxic thoughts and build up healthy thoughts—and in doing so, change your brain in a positive direction. This will result in peak thinking, happiness, and health. When applied daily within the correct time frames, it becomes a lifestyle of thinking that renews your mind, creates real change and freedom, and brings you ever closer to God.

I am always excited to share this theory and process with people because of the joy it brings to see the positive change it makes in the lives of those who truly apply it.

I demonstrated in my research in the early 1990s that the nonconscious metacognitive mind is much more powerful than the conscious cognitive mind. When you engage the nonconscious mind through deep thinking, you bring memories into the conscious mind in a vulnerable state, which means you can change them—or reconceptualize them. I also found that when the memories go back into the nonconscious mind, they are more complex. You have not simply added information, you have redesigned the memories—and this can go in a positive or negative direction. Scientifically, this is called "creative reconceptualization."[2]

As an individual, you *are* capable of making mental and emotional changes in your life. Through your thinking, you can actively re-create thoughts and, therefore, knowledge in your mind.

## God Is Revealing More Each Day

These research results have been reconfirmed recently, specifically related to post traumatic stress disorder (PTSD) trauma. Karim Nader, a professor at McGill University, has done groundbreaking research on memory that scientifically proves that we can renew our minds—more evidence of science catching up with the Bible. He shows that the emotional component of memories can be reconsolidated or changed when recalled into the conscious mind because they become vulnerable. So as a memory moves from the nonconscious mind to the conscious mind, it becomes vulnerable and susceptible to change.[3] This is precisely what I proposed and found in my research.

## My Documented Results

Some of my documented results using this deep-thinking, brain-engaging process were very exciting. My patients with closed-head injuries showed between 110 to 140 percent increase in their academic results. This academic increase started within approximately twenty-one days of starting my 5-Step Switch On Your Brain Learning Process. Furthermore, not only did it improve academic function, but intellectual, emotional, and social skills showed dramatic change as well. One patient in particular showed a better intellectual status, as evaluated on neuropsychological testing, after the accident than before. This means she increased her intelligence, according to the neuropsychologist, by up to 20 points post-accident when normally intellectual scores decrease by 20 to 30 points after a traumatic brain injury.

Her memory improvement was almost immediate and continued to improve dramatically over the twelve months of therapy. This improvement continued over time with her going on to further her studies and successfully moving into the work arena. Clinically, this patient became more organized and less confused, and she was perceived by her peers as being no different from them.

This is a major feat because statistical estimates suggest that only one third of patients who suffer traumatic brain injury might return to their previous lifestyle and gainful employment with traditional therapy. In contrast, the 5-Step Switch On Your Brain Learning Process, my nontraditional therapeutic approach, works on metacognitive and cognitive mind issues (see chap. 8), and the improvement in the metacognitive and cognitive mind issues carries over into intellect, emotions, and psychosocial functioning. Probably the most impactful is that the improvement carries over into everyday life and is therefore self-sustaining.

## We Can All Get Control of Our Minds

At the same time I was working with traumatic brain injury (TBI) patients, I also worked with students with learning problems as well as students who had no learning problems as such, but who wanted to improve their academic progress. My work also included adults pursuing further education and those in corporate life. In my doctoral research, I showed that significant changes in cognitive, academic, and psychosocial function happened in teachers and students alike when they applied my deep-thinking brain technique. Across the board, I was seeing these same kinds of results. I trained thousands of teachers and therapists in my 5-Step Switch On Your Brain Learning Process, and they have, in turn, reached thousands of students and report great changes.

### Put Your Mind to It

I even saw this happening in the most challenging of situations back in my home country of South Africa. For many years I worked with starving children who had literally not eaten for many days. In most cases they didn't have two loving parents at home because at least one if not both had either died of AIDS or had been murdered, and they lived in squalid conditions with more than a 70 percent chance of having been exposed to some form of physical, sexual, or mental abuse—yet they could not get enough of learning how to learn when I ran Switch On Your Brain courses in their schools.

Even though I was working through the medium of academics in these schools, the sessions became like church services when those brave children recognized that they could use their minds to rise above their circumstances, and that they could change their life with this incredible mind and brain God had given them. They saw learning as an exciting opportunity and wanted to be at school, despite the fact that there were often a hundred hungry, dirty, traumatized children squeezed into a classroom where we would have only one textbook to work from and one old-fashioned chalkboard. They were desperate to learn and sat for hours listening raptly and hardly moving, as though trying to absorb everything I was teaching into every fiber of their being. It was a privilege to be there with those magnificent minds dressed in rags, and this was where I learned some of my greatest lessons about the power of choice and deep, intellectual thought to change the mind.

### It's Not a Heavy Burden

Some researchers who visited Soweto, South Africa, where I worked for years, have compared these amazing children in Soweto to Harvard students, though you could not have two more different worlds.[4] Their results showed that 95 percent of the Soweto children said they loved schoolwork and learning; in comparison, about 80 percent (4 out of 5) of the Harvard students suffered from depression so debilitating they could not function.[5] This is shocking considering that Harvard has some of the brightest minds, magnificent facilities, and is mentioned often as the gold standard of education.

When you see choosing to change your mind and to learn as a heavy burden, you miss out on the opportunities in front of you. When you see choosing to change your mind and to learn as a wonderful privilege, suddenly you see the opportunities.

What I saw in the people I have worked with over the years, some of whom are described in the studies in earlier chapters and above, was a mindset that chose to change and excel. They chose not to allow their difficult life experience to block them. They *chose to change*. They chose not to succumb to the pressure nor to get stuck in a neutral position and settle for the status quo.

Do you want to choose to change? Choosing life is the mindset that brings renewal and revival. This is what I hope my 21-Day Brain Detox Plan will help you achieve.

## Chapter 9 Summary

1. You have to *choose* to have a controlled thought life and to be happy and healthy. Everyone can learn how to improve their thinking, learning, and intelligence.

2. We need to wire in positive thought networks that can fill us with the power to get us back on track (2 Tim. 1:7).

3. Even though the 5 Steps of the Switch on Your Brain Learning Process that are used daily in the 21-Day Brain Detox are based on rigorous science and the Word of

God, they are a simple tool to help bring peak happiness, thinking, and health not only into your life but also the lives of your loved ones.

4. To detox your thought life, you need to remember *it's your thinking that will actually change your brain.*

5. Science is catching up with the Bible daily.

6. If you put your mind to it, you can achieve what God says you can achieve.

7. You control your brain; your brain does not control you.

# 10

# How and Why the 21-Day Brain Detox Plan Works

The Switch On Your Brain 21-Day Brain Detox Plan technique is a rigorous, disciplined, daily routine that becomes a lifestyle of renewing your mind. It is a lifestyle of neuroplastically rewiring your nerve networks. It is driven by you, but led by the Holy Spirit. It gets you into a state of deep, intellectual, introspective self-reflection, activating all eight keys I described in part 1.

## Your Daily Routine

Once you have worked through this book and mastered the concepts (and take your time with this; it's worth not rushing through), your daily routine will take *seven to ten* minutes minimum, although some like to go longer. During this time you will be doing 5 steps, daily, for 21 days. These 5 steps are based on my research on the science of thought and the brain (see chapter 8) and are called the 5-Step Switch On Your Brain Learning Process.

You can do up to *seventeen* 21-Day Brain Detox Plan cycles per year.[1] Research shows that deep-thinking exercises repeated daily over a period of twenty-one days help create long-lasting change.

Your year can start whenever you want it to, so if you have picked up this book in September, for example, then you simply work through the book during September and then begin your year in October.

Who needs this? Everyone. As you have seen from the eight keys discussed in part 1, no one is exempt from mind issues. From the moment God created us with free will, we entered a realm of creative responsibility for our choices.

It is obviously a highly complex process, but I have simplified the Switch On Your Brain technique sequence into five steps:

1. Gather
2. Focused Reflection
3. Write
4. Revisit
5. Active Reach

## You Are Doing Your Own Brain Surgery

Each of these steps activates phenomenal and complex neurophysiology and neurobiology. So in essence, what you will be doing with the 5 steps is bringing the toxic thought into consciousness and then proceeding, over 21 days, to destroy it (see chap. 8). Mind controls matter, as we learned in part 1.

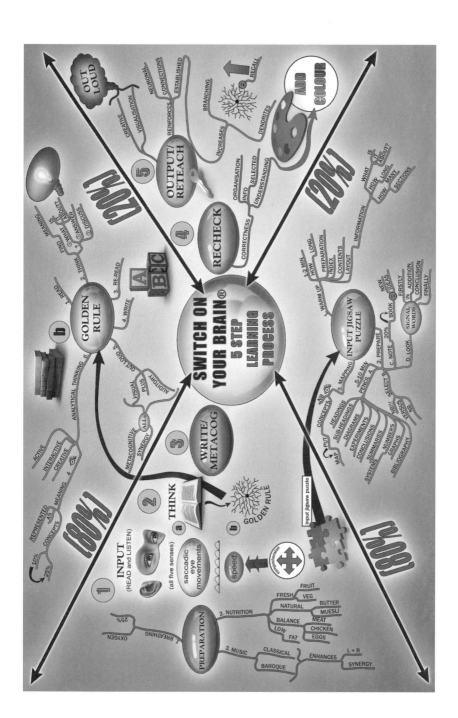

At the same time, you will be growing a healthy new thought to replace the toxic one, so you will be consciously and simultaneously building up healthy thoughts and tearing down toxic thoughts. You work on only *one* thought network each 21-day cycle, breaking down the toxic and simultaneously building up the healthy.

## You Can Repeat the Cycle

You may repeat a cycle if you feel you haven't fully dealt with the issue. Many times we start working through something only to discover the root issue a few days in. That's fine; just focus in on the root issue for the rest of the 21 days and then redo the cycle. Twenty-one days is just the minimum time needed to build the neural network.[2]

What this means is that it takes repeated updating or rethinking through information in a sequenced way for it to take root and form a stable memory. If this reinforcement does not take place over the 21 days, then the newly found neural network will decay in less than a month. If you don't use the memory, the proteins it is made from will denature and the memory will disassemble. Wherever there is more thinking activity, there will be more wiring. Whatever you think about the most will grow, because thinking stimulates the genetic expression required to make proteins. Every hour the connections are doubling.[3]

You may also just feel at the end of the cycle that the toxic thought was so dominant or strong that it warrants working on it another 21 days. Sometimes there is a lot of guilt and condemnation or "I can't" mindsets that can keep you from progressing. These mindsets alone require a 21-day brain detox before the next issue can be tackled.

## Pay More Attention to the New, Healthy Memory

This is why it is so important to build up the new healthy memory and pay more attention to it rather than to the toxic memory you are breaking down: Repeated replaying is central to the process of creating durable, long-term memories. And remember, this works in both the negative and positive direction.

As you move through the five steps and into deep, focused reflection, your brain will have moments of insight that are accompanied by bursts of high frequency gamma waves in the brain.[4] These create an ideal mindset for learning and integration across the brain. Neurons have their own rhythmic activity, almost like an internal chatter, and changes in these fluctuations underlie how we perceive things.[5] It is our choice to pay attention that influences this internal chatter in a positive or negative direction. You want as much of this happening over the 21 days as possible because it will enhance your effectiveness. We need to be almost obsessive in our desire to change, to "Be perfect, therefore, as your heavenly Father is perfect" (Matt. 5:48 NIV).

## So Many Good Things Are Happening

The brain is always learning how to learn, always changing. As you use the 5-Step Switch On Your Brain Learning Process through the 21 days you are influencing so many good things to happen. Here are just a few. When you think deeply and are learning, BDNF (brain derived neurotrophic factor) is released to consolidate the connections between neurons to enhance recall in the future. This BDNF also promotes increase in the fatty substance called myelin, which insulates the nerves. This is a good thing, because increased myelination means faster thinking and better memory. As you start paying attention and focusing your thinking, BDNF is released, and this in turn increases attention by activating the nucleus basalis. And when the nucleus basalis is turned on, the brain becomes extremely plastic and ready to change, build, and rewire—and therefore, renew.[6]

## The Work Doesn't End at 21 Days

At the end of the 21-day cycle, the toxic thought is gone and the new healthy thought is like a "tiny new plant" that will need nurturing to grow. Our *thinking* is that nurturing. This means that if you don't practice using it, it will not be properly automatized (see chap. 8), and it is very possible that your mind will shift back to regrowing that toxic thought.

To avoid this you make a conscious effort to practice using the new thought as much as you can until you reach automatization. Automatization means that particular way of thinking or reacting embedded in the new thought tree has become an automatic part of you; you do it driven by the nonconscious mind, not the conscious mind. So, to make sure that you have automatized the new healthy memory, research shows you will need to consciously practice using it daily for at least two more 21-day cycles, or 63 days total.[7] Please continue to consciously keep practicing using the new habit until you feel comfortable—which can even sometimes take between 84–154 days of consciously using the new healthy thought. The point is that the duration or automatization of the habit formation is likely to differ based on what you are trying to do and, of course, the uniqueness of who you are as a person. As long as you continue *doing*—which I call an "active reach," the fifth step that you do each day—consistently in a given situation, the healthy new way of thinking, the healthy "habit," will form.

## Bumps, Lollipops, and Mushrooms

In the brain, automatization physically looks like lots more tree branches that are thick and well established, with many branches interconnecting with other thought networks. And if you could zoom in closely to the connections the branches grow from, you would see little things called *spines*. These spines change shape, from a bump at around 7 days, to a lollipop shape at around 14 days, to a mushroom shape at around 21 days as the thought becomes stronger. This is because the proteins change progressively by day 21, with peak changes being at 7 and 14 days, to become self-sustaining proteins, which are like a long-term memory. This applies in both the negative and positive direction—this is the concept of the plastic paradox I spoke of earlier. And even a long-term memory can be broken down. If, after wiring out a toxic thought, you have stopped using the healthy new thought and revert back to the toxic thought, you reverse the process you went through in the first place, breaking down the healthy thought and rebuilding the toxic thought. This is why we need to make a choice to be alert, practicing the presence of God by sharpening our conscience and listening to our intuition. This is what creates a lifestyle of renewing the mind.

So at the end of the 21 days, you integrate the new healthy thought into your lifestyle, into your repertoire of reactions to life so that you keep strengthening that reaction. It can take anywhere from three to four 21-day cycles to automatize

## A Neuron with Dendrites, Showing Bumps, Lollipops, and Umbrellas

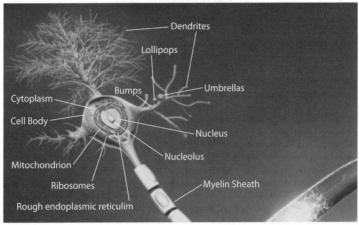

the new healthy thought pattern and to make sure the toxic thought doesn't grow back.[8] A lot also depends on the individual, the thought pattern you are detoxing, and the healthy replacement pattern you are building. So for some thoughts it might take one 21-day cycle, and for other thoughts it might take more, as I explained earlier.

### The 21-Day Brain Detox Plan Is a Deliberate Practice

The best way to change, learn, and build memory meaningfully is through deliberate and disciplined practice. This is not mindless repetition. The five steps of the Switch On Your Brain technique in the 21-Day Brain Detox Plan include deliberate, conscious setting of goals, obtaining immediate feedback, and concentrating as much on the process as on the outcome. The 21-Day Brain Detox Plan will work best when you set the challenge just beyond the edge of your comfort zone; a challenge is good for you.[9] We are designed as deeply intelligent beings and our minds and brains respond to and rise up to challenge. In fact, they get better.

You are made from God's perfectness, but it is up to you to create your expertise in life. God gives us the blueprint, but we need to choose to make it happen.

The point is that you are playing to win and you don't give up. "I press on toward the goal to win the prize for which God has called me heavenward in Christ Jesus" (Phil. 3:14 NIV). As you go through this process, you will be fulfilling what God calls us to do in Romans 12:2, "renewing" the mind, and in Matthew 5:48, "Be perfect, just as your Father in heaven is perfect." In the next five chapters I will explain each of the five steps of my Switch On Your Brain technique. It is necessary to get a deep understanding of each of these steps so you use them properly on a daily basis. If you skip a step or only sort of use the step, the changes you create will also be "sort of" and not effective.

You will see questions interspersed in the text—please stop to take a moment to answer the questions because they will help you experience and understand the Switch On Your Brain process much more deeply, and it will make it easier to apply the 21-Day Brain Detox Plan. The questions help you start understanding how to get into the mindset that will increase your chance of success.

## Chapter 10 Summary

1. The 21-Day Brain Detox Plan is a deliberate, disciplined, and rigorous renewing of the mind lifestyle, not a one-time activity.
2. Your daily routine will take seven to ten minutes minimum, although some like to go longer.

3. You will be doing approximately seventeen 21-Day Brain Detox Plan cycles per year.

4. Each day you do my 5-Step Switch On Your Brain Learning Process for the seven to ten minutes.

5. Over the 21 days, you are breaking down the toxic thought and building up the healthy replacement memory.

6. It takes 21 days for certain protein changes to happen in the brain for the new memory to become self-sustaining and for the old memory to be broken down.

7. By approximately day 7 the protein connection holding the memory in place is a bump shape; by approximately day 14 it is a lollipop shape; and by approximately day 21 it is a mushroom shape.

8. You need to repeat the 21-day cycle for up to three more times for it to become automatized.

9. *Automatization* means it is in your nonconscious controlling the conscious thinking that precedes what you do.

# 11

## Gather

*Step 1*

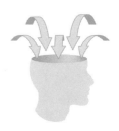

You have to develop disciplined thought lives, and part of that is increasing your awareness of what you are allowing into your mind. The *gather* step is, therefore, all about becoming aware of all the signals that are coming into your mind from the external environment through the five senses and understanding the internal environment of your mind. So as you answer the questions in this section, you are focusing on developing *awareness*, which means you are starting the process of bringing those rogue thoughts into captivity.

### The Signals Come from Two Sources

These signals come from two sources: (1) the external environment that comes in through the five senses, electromagnetic and quantum signals, and (2) the thoughts deep in the nonconscious metacognitive part of your mind (your memories).

Let me explain what I mean. Perhaps, as you read this, you have some of your favorite music playing in the background. You might be sitting in a comfortable chair, smelling a scented candle while savoring a piece of fruit. If you are in this idyllic setting, all five of your senses—sight, sound, smell, touch, and taste—will be your link between the external world and the internal world of your mind.

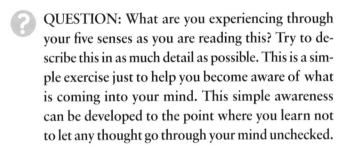

QUESTION: What are you experiencing through your five senses as you are reading this? Try to describe this in as much detail as possible. This is a simple exercise just to help you become aware of what is coming into your mind. This simple awareness can be developed to the point where you learn not to let any thought go through your mind unchecked.

As we move on with this section, there is a lot of brain information. Take your time and just enjoy how intricately God has made you. And please remember, you are brilliant and intelligent and totally capable of understanding because you are made in his image (Gen. 1:26).

## The Signals Enter the Brain

This incoming information then travels through some astonishing brain structures (some of which include the thalamus, insula, and basal ganglia) that flavor, enrich, and distribute the information all along the way. You think with groups of brain areas (circuits and columns), not with single brain areas. So once the information enters the brain, it is a signal that creates major cascading, intrinsic (inside your brain) activity. The circuits and columns around the basal ganglia (deep down inside the middle of the brain), for example, get

# Inside the Brain

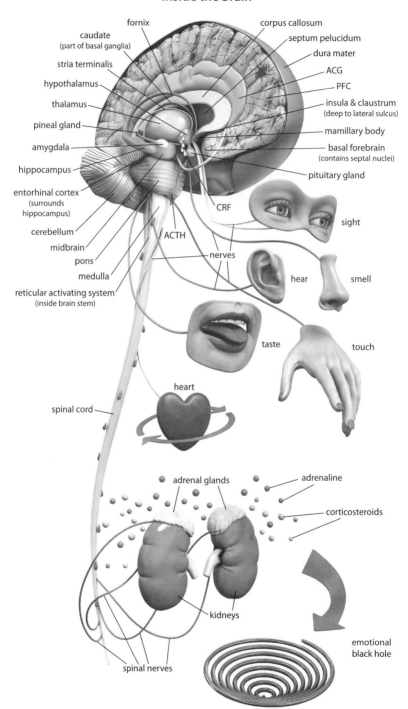

fornix

corpus callosum

caudate
(part of basal ganglia)

septum pelucidum

stria terminalis

dura mater

hypothalamus

ACG

thalamus

PFC

pineal gland

insula & claustrum
(deep to lateral sulcus)

amygdala

mamillary body

hippocampus

basal forebrain
(contains septal nuclei)

entorhinal cortex
(surrounds
hippocampus)

pituitary gland

CRF

cerebellum

sight

midbrain

ACTH

pons

nerves

medulla

reticular activating system
(inside brain stem)

hear

smell

taste

touch

heart

spinal cord

adrenal glands

adrenaline

corticosteroids

kidneys

emotional
black hole

spinal nerves

the brain into a state of expectation as preparation to build the new, incoming information. Part of this activity is the movement of thoughts (existing memories), linked in some way to the incoming information, moving from the nonconscious metacognitive level to the conscious cognitive level (see chap. 8 to remind yourself of these concepts).

### "Magic Trees of the Mind" Golgi Stain

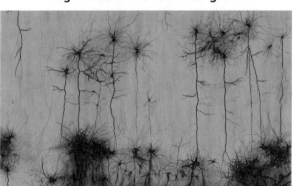

These thoughts in your brain look like trees in a forest. And as the signals sweep through these trees like a wind, research shows they will activate around four to seven[1] thought trees (memories) that will then move into the conscious, and you will become aware of them (see chap. 8). I call this the "breeze through the trees."

 QUESTION: What thoughts are bubbling up into your conscious mind right at this moment? Focus in and see how many there are.

### Thoughts Have an Emotional Component

When you think, you *also feel*. This is because thoughts have an emotional component in addition to the information, or

160

what the actual memory is about. This means that when you bring a thought into consciousness, you also bring up the attached emotion. When the thought along with its emotions bubble up into the conscious mind, you *feel* the emotions.

So there is a difference between emotions and feelings; every thought has *emotions* as part of its structure, and they are stored in the nonconscious mind. When the thoughts move into the conscious mind, we *feel* the emotions of the thoughts.

## Attitude

Attitude is a *state of mind*—a thought plus its attached emotions—and it influences what you say and do.

If the attitude that is activated is negative, then the emotional response will naturally be a negative or stressful feeling. If the attitude is positive, the feeling will be peaceful. The truth is that your attitude will be revealed no matter how much you try to hide it.

 QUESTION: Can you determine the attitude of the thoughts that are currently moving through your conscious mind? Try to focus in on the feelings they are generating and describe them in as much detail as possible. How does your mind feel? How does your body feel?

## Thoughts Can't Be Hidden; Attitudes Aren't Harmless

Your attitudes—positive or negative—not only can't be hidden from others, but they also have a profound impact on your own brain and body. You can refer back to chapter 7 for a reminder of how this works.

When a thought, plus its emotions (attitudes), moves into the conscious mind, it produces a signal. The hypothalamus (see image), which does many amazing things—one of which is to respond to our emotional state of mind or our attitude—responds to this signal.

## The Hypothalamus Responds

Part of what the hypothalamus does is alert the rest of the brain to release chemicals like serotonin and glutamate to help with the process of building a new memory. The endocrine system is a collection of glands and organs that mostly produce and regulate your hormones. And the hypothalamus is often referred to as the "brain" of the endocrine system, controlling things like thirst, hunger, body temperature, and the body's response to your emotional life. The hypothalamus is also like a pulsating heart responding to your emotions and thought life, greatly impacting how you function emotionally and intellectually.

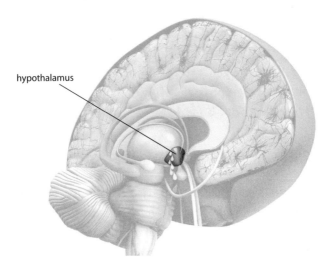

hypothalamus

This means that if you are anxious or worried about something, the hypothalamus will respond by releasing more chemicals than it should. This in turn causes the pituitary to release too many chemicals, and the result is neurochemical chaos. So instead of being focused in our thinking, we have chaotic and foggy thinking.

The endocrine system secretes the hormones responsible for organizing the trillions of cells in your body to deal with focus and learning. Negative, toxic thoughts have the opposite effect, shifting your body's focus to protection and survival, thus reducing your ability to process and think with wisdom or grow healthy thoughts.

However, if you change your attitude and determine to apply God's excellent advice not to worry, the hypothalamus will cause the secretion of chemicals that facilitate the feeling of peace, and the rest of the brain will respond by secreting the correct formula of neurotransmitters—chemicals that transmit electrical impulses—for thought-building and clear thinking.

 QUESTION: Do the thoughts in your conscious mind at this moment make you feel peace or worry? Be aware of how your body feels. Are you tensing your shoulders? Is there an adrenaline rush going through your body?

Although you may not be able to control your environment all of the time, you can control how it affects your brain.

## You Can Control How the Signals Affect Your Brain

How? The incoming information is still in a temporary state. It has not yet lodged itself into your memory, or become a part of your spirit, which defines who you are. You can choose to reject the presently activated thoughts and the incoming information, or you can let the information make its way into your mind, soul, and your spirit, eventually subsiding in your nonconscious and becoming automatized, dominating who you are. Even though you can't always control your circumstances, you can make fundamental choices that will help you control your reaction to your circumstances and keep toxic input out of your brain.

> **QUESTION:** Do you feel like a victim of or a victor over what is swarming through your mind at the moment from the external and internal signals?

## Brain Structures and Circuits That Help You Make Good Choices

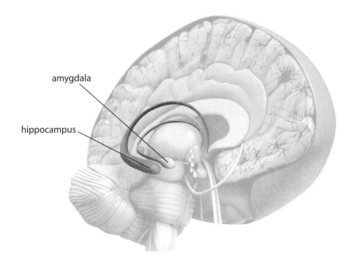

The amygdala and hippocampus, and their connected circuits, can help you make good choices. The amygdala deals with the passionate, perceptual emotions attached to incoming thoughts and all the thoughts already in your head. The hippocampus deals with memory and motivation.

This is where you consciously step up to center stage; you need to choose, and decide whether or not these incoming thoughts will become part of who you are. Let's look more closely at how you control this decision to accept or reject information.

 **QUESTION: Did you know you are able to accept or reject the thoughts flowing through your mind?**

### The Amygdala: Perceptual Library

The amygdala, a double almond–shaped structure located in your brain, is designed to keep you emotionally alert. When you become toxic in your thinking, it steps up to protect you from any threat to your body and mind—such as danger or stress. It puts the passion behind the punch of memory formation by influencing another structure that is very important to memory formation, the hippocampus, enabling you to give more focused attention to your existing memories. The amygdala is basically designed to deal with positive love-based emotions like joy and happiness, but it doesn't work as well when you are in a negative state of mind.

### The Thalamus Acts Like a Transmitter Station

The thalamus (deep in the middle of the brain) functions like a transmitter station, alerting the amygdala of any incoming information from the five senses. How does it do this?

The amygdala functions like a library, storing the emotional perceptions that occur each time a thought is built. In other words, every time you build a memory, you activate emotions. The endocrine system in the brain has to release the correct

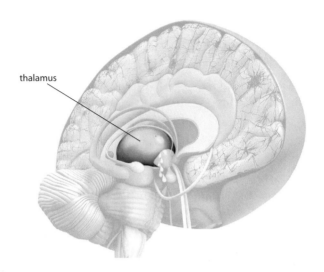

thalamus

chemicals—the molecules of emotion and information—necessary to build healthy or toxic memories. Because the amygdala is in constant communication with the hypothalamus, which secretes chemicals in response to your thought life, you are able to feel your body's reaction to your thoughts. These physical reactions—rapid heartbeat and adrenaline rushes—force you to decide whether to accept or reject the information, basing your decision on how you feel physically.

To help you even more, the amygdala has lines of communication connected to the frontal lobe, which controls reasoning, decision-making, analyzing, and strategizing—all executive-level functions. This connection enables you to balance the emotions you physically experience in your body and allows you to react reasonably. Here is the exciting part: At this moment you can choose *not* to think about this issue anymore, and those temporary thoughts will disappear.

 QUESTION: You do not have to be dominated by your perceptual library—in other words your emotions. Do you feel dominated by your feelings that have arisen out of the thoughts active in your mind?

### The Hippocampus: Memory Converter

If you don't manage to stop thinking about the issue, however, all the information, including the awakened toxic or nontoxic attitude, will flow into a sea horse–shaped structure called the hippocampus.

The hippocampus is a sort of clearinghouse for thoughts. It classifies incoming information as having either short- or long-term importance and files it accordingly, converting temporary thoughts into permanent thoughts that become part of who you are (a lot of this happens at night while you are sleeping). To do this, the hippocampus has to work with the central hub of the brain—a group of structures with circuits that integrate all the activated memories and work with the hippocampus to convert information into your permanent memory storage.

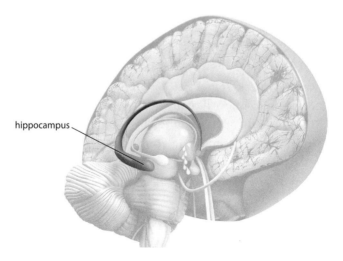

hippocampus

This is where you begin some serious reflection in order to make some life-changing decisions.

 QUESTION: Ask yourself, "Do I want this information to be a part of me?"

### Stress

A good point to remember is that toxic memories create the negative stage two and negative stage three of stress. Stage one of stress is good and keeps you alert and focused. Stage two and three are normal stress gone wrong.

The hippocampus is extremely vulnerable to stress because it is rich in stress hormone receptors that are normally used to reinforce memories. These receptors are like tiny doorways on cells that receive chemical information. For these brain cells, excessive stress is almost like an explosion, causing the hippocampus to lose cells and shrink. This affects the communication between the hippocampus and the central circuits of the brain, keeping it from building new good thoughts (memories) as well as causing memory loss. This is seen a lot in depression, Alzheimer's, dementias, and other neuropsychiatric disorders.

 QUESTION: Toxic thoughts are the result of bad choices. Stress stages two and three are your body's reaction to toxic thoughts. Can you feel the stress reaction—heart pounding, adrenaline pumping, or muscles tensing up in your body?

### Chapter 11 Summary

1. Sensory information flows into the brain through the five senses.

2. Existing memories in the nonconscious are activated.

3. This activates memories to move from nonconscious to the conscious mind and attitudes are invoked.

4. The hypothalamus responds to the attitude by releasing chemicals necessary for memory building and emotions.

5. This activates the amygdala to recall linked emotional perceptions and to start building in new emotional perceptions.

6. All this information enters the hippocampus, which is involved in converting short-term memory to long-term memory.

7. All this electromagnetic, chemical, and quantum physics activity moves to the front of the brain.

Let's move to the reflection stage and see how the hippocampus works with the central hub circuits of the brain in building thoughts.

# 12

# Focused Reflection

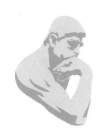

*Step 2*

It is always fun to see science catching up with the Bible, as we discussed in part 1. Focused reflection is an example of this. It is an ancient biblical principle most of us know. But it is also the current rage in neuroscience, and there are hundreds of studies with headlines like

"Mindfulness Meditation May Relieve Chronic Inflammation"[1]

"Evidence Supports Health Benefits of 'Mindfulness-Based Practices'"[2]

"Breast Cancer Survivors Benefit from Practicing Mindfulness-Based Stress Reduction"[3]

"Don't Worry, Be Happy: Understanding Mindfulness Meditation"[4]

"Mindfulness Meditation Training Changes Brain Structure in Eight Weeks"[5]

You get the idea.

## It Always Boils Down to One Thing

Although a lot of these studies talk about Eastern meditation techniques, what it boils down to every time is deep, intellectual, disciplined thinking with attention regulation, thinking, body awareness, emotion regulation, and a sense of self that changes the brain positively. Consequently, people gain health, happiness—and peace—exactly the instruction and consequence of Philippians 4:8: "Finally, brothers and sisters, whatever is true, whatever is noble, whatever is right, whatever is pure, whatever is lovely, whatever is admirable— if anything is excellent or praiseworthy—think about such things" (NIV). In fact, throughout the book of Proverbs we are instructed to gain wisdom and meditate on knowledge until we understand.

## Getting Out of a Toxic-Thinking Block

If you are going to get out of any toxic-thinking block, you need to think, understand, and apply the wisdom you gain.[6]

Thankfully, you have all the structures and physiological processes at your disposal to do this. Neuroplasticity (key 3) and quantum physics (key 7) are for your benefit and can help you enjoy every day. Don't forget that, as a neuroplastician, you can do your own brain surgery. This means no thought should ever be allowed to control you (see chaps. 1 and 2).

So once you have gone through the whole gathering awareness step above—which disciplines you to be careful of what's going into your brain as well as what is coming out from inside—then you need to go deep and focus your reflection. As you apply keys 4 and 5 in this step (catch your thoughts and enter into directed rest), an incredible change happens in your brain. Let's look at some of the technical side interspersed with some focused questions to help you digest the science.

Just a quick reminder here: Each of these 5 steps that you do daily for 21 days are simple, yet there are profound parallel and simultaneous neurophysiological things going on in your brain that are so marvelous you cannot help but be one who "admires God's work," as Thomas More put it. So don't let yourself get overwhelmed by the science; instead, look at it with fascination and admiration of our gracious God. Science is pure evidence of grace.

## The Rush to the Front of the Brain

After the gathering stage, the electromagnetic signals—your thinking and those existing memories that have been brought into consciousness—speed through the hippocampus, moving toward the front of the brain—the basal forebrain and orbitofrontal cortex, which are behind the inside corners of

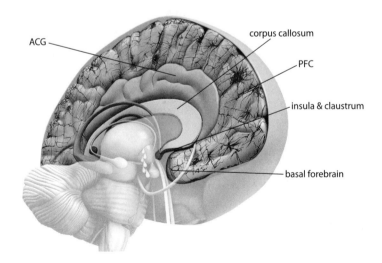

your eyes and above your eyebrows respectively. The information flows through in the hippocampus for twenty-four to forty-eight hours, constantly being amplified each time it cycles to the front.

### Free Will

The amplification sets in motion a delightful string of events so magnificent that it can only reflect the work of your Creator. This string of events is your free will and decision-making ability, a true gift. (Before you go on, please look back at the summaries of keys 1, 2, 3, and 7.)

### The Thought Becomes Vulnerable to Change

This amplification means the thought is conscious and becomes "labile," which means it is unstable and changeable. In fact, it must change (see chap. 3). The science of thought demands that change must occur either by reinforcing the thought as it is or by changing some or all of it.

The memory cannot sink back as part of your attitude into your nonconscious mind without being changed in some way. This is marvelous news for you, but it also emphasizes the responsibility you need to take for your thought life. No thought is harmless, nor does it stay the same—it constantly changes. As I said in part 1, you are constantly changing the landscape of your brain moment by moment. You are a thinking, creative being—quite brilliant.

 QUESTION: Now that you are aware that thoughts are unstable and changeable when they are in your conscious cognitive mind, can you focus on one in particular and experimenting with changing it?

## When You Think, You Change

This constant change means that the deeper you think, the more change you can make. This change is real and happens via electromagnetic and quantum forces as well as neurotransmitters activating genetic expression and protein synthesis (see chaps. 2 and 3).

As a reminder, proteins are made and used to grow new branches to hold your thoughts. So if you don't get rid of the thought, you reinforce it. This is phenomenal because science confirms that you can choose with your free will to interfere with genetic expression, which is protein synthesis (chap. 2). If you say you can't or won't, this decision will actually cause protein synthesis and change in your brain into "I can't" or "I won't." Remember: mind controls matter (chap. 1). Now "bringing into captivity every thought" (2 Cor. 10:5 KJV) becomes a lot more important. Thoughts are constantly remodeled by the "renewing of your mind" (Rom. 12:2 NIV).

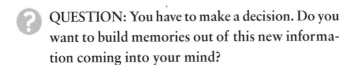

QUESTION: You have to make a decision. Do you want to build memories out of this new information coming into your mind?

When you do this, as you saw in chapters 2 and 3, you actually change the physical structure—neuroplasticity—of your brain. This is because thinking causes important neurotransmitters—chemicals in the brain that carry electrical impulses—to flow. These neurotransmitters plus electromagnetic and quantum activity cause changes deep inside the cell, affecting genetic expression and protein synthesis, as I have described earlier.

## Imagining Builds Physical Thoughts

Research has shown that mental practice—imagination, visualization, deep thought, and reflection—produces the same physical changes in the brain as would physically carrying out the same imagined processes. We see this principle in the Bible: "Nothing they have imagined they can do will be impossible for them" (Gen. 11:6 AMP). Brain scans show that the parts of the brain activated by action are the same parts of the brain activated by simply thinking about an action. This sheds new depths of understanding for the Scripture, "Faith is the substance of things hoped for, the evidence of things not seen" (Heb. 11:1).

Rehearsing things mentally is a great everyday example of how you can think and more deeply reflect on daily actions, because each time you do this, you change the memory. For example, if a surgeon is about to perform an operation, he first mentally rehearses each precise step, as would an athlete before a game or a student about to take an exam. As you mentally rehearse it, the newly built memory becomes increasingly stronger and begins to grow more connections to neighboring nerve cells, integrating that thought into other thought patterns. This leads to automatization, which I spoke about in chapter 8.

 **QUESTION: Have you ever found yourself rehearsing something over and over for days on end, almost like you couldn't get it out of your head? How did that make you feel?**

A healthy thought and a toxic thought can both be built with mental rehearsal. But you can tear toxic strongholds down by choosing to bring the thought into conscious awareness for analysis and then changing it through repentance and forgiveness—which causes protein synthesis—and replacing it with the correct information, using Philippians 4:8 or a similar Scripture guideline.

 **QUESTION: How do you tear down the toxic stronghold?**

## The Contribution of the Heart

When talking about thinking, free will, and understanding, you need to also consider the exciting contribution the heart makes to thinking and decision-making. Your heart is not just a pump; it helps with decision-making and choices, acting like a checking station for all the emotions generated by the flow of chemicals from thoughts. In fact, every single cell is connected to your heart and, because your heart responds to and is controlled by your brain, every single cell in your body is affected by your thoughts.

Your heart is in constant communication with your brain and the rest of your body, checking the accuracy and integrity of your thought life. As you are about to make a decision, your heart pops in a quiet word of advice. It is well worth listening to this advice, because when you listen to your heart, it secretes the ANF (atrial natriuretic factor)—a hormone produced by the heart that regulates blood pressure and can give you a feeling of peace.

 **QUESTION: What role does the heart play in focused reflection?**

## Expertise

When you think deeply to understand, you go beyond just storing facts and answers to storing key concepts and strategies

# Inside the Brain

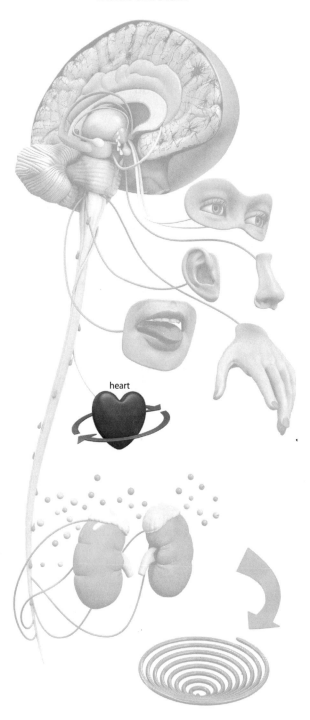

that can help you come up with your own answers. These thoughts have been consolidated and stabilized sufficiently so that you have immediate access to them. When this happens, you have achieved a level of expertise. But this can happen in a negative or positive direction, with all the contributing effects. You should be aiming for that which you were naturally designed—deep, intellectual, nontoxic thought (Matthew 5:48). Focused reflection helps with this process, but for protein synthesis to consolidate, stabilize, and become part of you, repetition and rehearsal in frequent, spaced intervals is necessary. The next three stages in thought formation—writing, revisit, and active reach—show you how to take advantage of this to stabilize your protein synthesis or bring your memory back up again to retranscribe or change it.

## Chapter 12 Summary

1. Focused thinking is specifically focusing on one thought with its interconnections.
2. It is a directed and deep, intellectual process.
3. It is a disciplined way of thinking that has the elements of attention regulation, controlling raging, and preventing chaotic thoughts from moving through the mind.
4. It includes body awareness, emotion regulation, and sense of self that changes the brain positively.
5. Keys 1 through 8 really kick in at this point.
6. Huge activity in the center and front of the brain happens when we focus our thinking.
7. Neuroplasticity is dominant because, as you focus your thinking, you are starting to redesign your brain.

# 13

## Write

*Step 3*

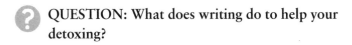

Your brain writes through genetic expression, so when you write things down on paper or type into your computer or iPad or whatever gadget you use, you are mirroring this process. Writing down your thoughts is important in the Switch On Your Brain technique because the actual process of writing consolidates the memory and adds clarity to what you have been thinking about. It helps you better see the area that needs to be detoxed by allowing you to see your nonconscious and conscious thoughts in a visual way. It is almost like putting your brain on paper.

**QUESTION: What does writing do to help your detoxing?**

The basal ganglia, the cerebellum, and the motor cortex are involved in this process. Let's talk about the basal ganglia first.

### The Industrious Basal Ganglia

Nestling between the cerebral cortex (on the outside of the brain) and the midbrain (in both the left and right hemispheres)

181

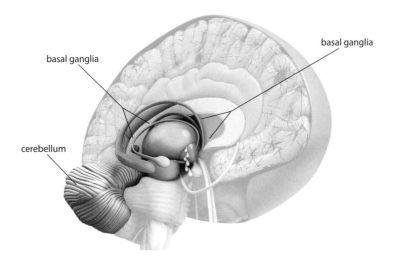

are intricate bundles of neurological networks that are interconnected with the cerebral cortex. These bundles are the basal ganglia. The basal ganglia also put their imprint on the process of thinking and learning by helping the hippocampus, frontal lobe, and corpus callosum turn thought and emotion into immediate action.

Remember, all the parts of the brain work together in harmony; the process never involves just one structure alone. The basal ganglia do this by helping to ensure the memory gets built into the trees of the cerebral cortex. They also smooth out fine motor actions and set the idle rate for anxiety. Together with the motor cortex of the brain, the cerebellum helps you write down the information you have just understood. The cerebellum also helps with cognitive fluency, which is the ability to flow through a thought process smoothly as you evaluate the options.

Obviously, all your brain structures become very involved in the writing process because writing is a complex cognitive and metacognitive process requiring deep thinking. For example, the structures in the frontal lobe become highly active in the thinking and decision-making part of writing; the temporal lobe and hippocampus become involved in calling up existing memories; the emotional parts of every activated thought generate feelings; and the structures in the middle of the brain dealing with emotional perceptions work harder, just to mention a few things. The complexity God has designed is beautiful.

 QUESTION: What do the basal ganglia help with?

## How to Write Your Thoughts

How you write down your thoughts is very important because there are ways of writing down information that work more effectively with your brain processes than traditional linear and one-color note taking. My workbook and DVD series called *Switch On Your Brain*[1] provides ideas on how to be brain-compatible when you are writing.

I always encourage anyone who keeps a thought journal to be creative with their notes. I also encourage anyone moving through the process of detoxifying thoughts to be playful with their thought journal. Don't limit yourself to just writing in straight lines. If there are word associations or groupings that seem natural as you focus on information, group those on a page. Draw a picture or diagram to go along with that thought expression. Add color or texture. Pour out the impressions in your mind onto the page.

## The Metacog

When I am helping students develop their learning and retention skills, I teach them a method I've developed called *Metacog*. The name might seem a little odd, but the process is fascinating.

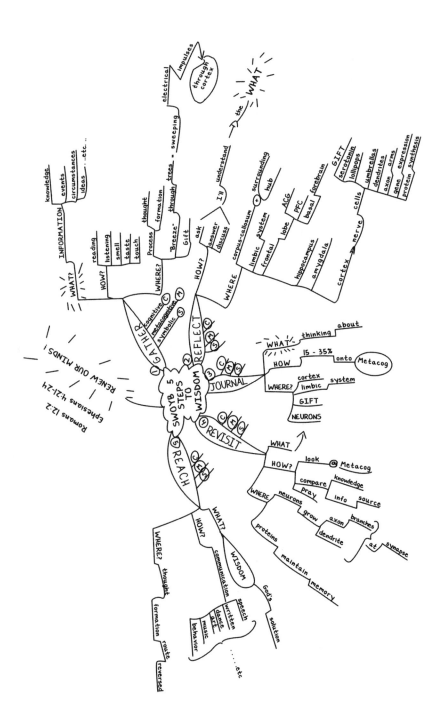

It is simple: Group patterns that radiate from a central point. Each pattern linked to the central point creates a branch. Then continue to develop each of the branches by linking more detailed patterns. The process can continue until you have explored every nuance of your thought.

This method of pouring out your thoughts encourages both sides of the brain to work together to integrate the two perspectives of thought—the left side of the brain looks at information from the detail to the big picture and the right side of the brain from the big picture to the detail.

For full understanding to take place—which will result in the conversion of short-term memory to long-term memory—both perspectives of thought need to come together. So a Metacog is a way of seeing your thoughts on paper and evaluating the way you think and what you are thinking about. It is a great way of following your thought patterns so you can detox your thought life.

## Chapter 13 Summary

1. The actual process of writing consolidates thoughts (memory).
2. Writing adds clarity to what you have been thinking about.
3. Writing helps you better see the area that needs to be detoxed by allowing you to see your nonconscious and conscious thoughts in a visual way.
4. Keep a thought journal.
5. Pour your thoughts out and only sort them in the next step—the revisit.

# 14

## Revisit

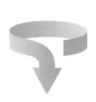

*Step 4*

R evisiting what you have written will be a revealing
process. This is exciting as well because it is a pro-
gressive "moving-forward" step; you revisit where
you are and look at how to make change happen.

After you have gathered awareness and done your focused
reflection and writing, you will have stimulated major neuroplastic activity, putting your brain in a highly active and
dynamic state for marvelous and positive change. This is the
perfect state to be in to rewire.

This step is all about you wiring in what changes you want.
You get to design your new healthy thought to replace the
toxic thought you want to get rid of. It's all about redesigning, reorganizing, and re-creating the specific thought you
are working on.

### Thoughts Become Plastic Enough to Be Redesigned

Earlier I explained that when thoughts are activated and
pushed into the conscious mind, they enter a labile state—
meaning they can be altered. When a memory is in this plastic

### Healthy Memory: Adapted Graphic Sketch

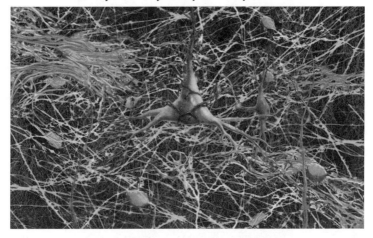

### Toxic Memory: Adapted Graphic Sketch

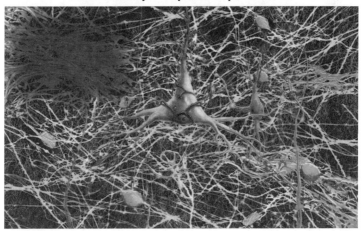

state, it can be modified, toned down, or retranscribed and reconceptualized by interfering with protein synthesis—an important molecular process in thought building. This is where you do some serious brain surgery (see chap. 3).

This is exciting, because once the thought is in the conscious mind after the gather, focused reflection, and writing you can redesign the thought and change it or keep it the same but make it stronger. You choose. Obviously, if you are doing the 21-Day Brain Detox Plan, you have chosen to change the negative, toxic thoughts.

God builds into the science of thought this amazing ability to renew our minds, which in turn rewires the brain. This means that each time a thought dominates your conscious mind, you can do something with it. You are not a victim of your biology; you can control your reactions to events and circumstances. You can choose to keep your thinking the same or change it. Either way, protein synthesis happens. The toxic memory will either be changed or be strengthened. This process is the major role of the revisit stage.

 QUESTION: How can thoughts be redesigned?

### How to Redesign Thoughts

In the revisit, you evaluate what you have written down and work out what the healthy new thought you want to build is going to be. You work out the way forward, a little at a time. Remember, you have twenty-one days to do this, so don't try to do it all in one day. Visualize what you want the end result to be, but get there in 21 days.

Not only do you have the opportunity to examine your thoughts on paper, but you have the opportunity to rethink through your reaction to the information—evaluating how toxic the thought is and then retranscribing it to be a healthy and strong part of your memory library.

By consciously becoming aware of your thought life you are retranscribing and changing your underlying neuronal networks. You need to uncover the toxic thoughts that create such powerful internal conflicts in your mind and that are capable of causing such radical electrochemical imbalances that, when taken to the extreme, cause parts of yourself to be cut off from the rest of you. While gather, focused reflection, and writing are hugely instrumental in this retranscribing and rewiring process, revisiting is a self-reflective process (see chap. 5) that has the purpose of getting free from the internal conflicts with positive planning of the way out. It is a constructive step that takes you through the problem, and it is cumulative. This means you need to think deeply and apply all the keys, which takes twenty-one days for the kind of depth in thinking that results in change. So you don't have to solve everything on day one—in fact, that would not be wise.

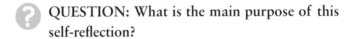 **QUESTION: What is the main purpose of this self-reflection?**

In revisiting, you are not only looking at how you go about dealing with your circumstances, but you are also thinking through your reactions again, evaluating the toxicity levels, and retranscribing them. This is a positive, looking-for-the-solution step. It feels safe because you are working out the way forward.

This is where the Bible is so perfect as a guide, because it lays out all the correct management principles for toxicity. At this revisit stage, if you discover you are a worrier, the Scripture in Matthew 6:25, which instructs us to not worry about tomorrow, is a good verse for you to apply.

So, if you line up your revisit with the principles outlined in God's Word instead of worldly psychology, you have a foolproof method for doing the right thing.

## Chapter 14 Summary

1. The revisit step is a moving-forward step during which you are working out solutions and ways to overcome.
2. This is when you evaluate where you have come from and where you are going.
3. You also have the opportunity to think through your reactions again, evaluating the toxicity levels, and reorganizing, redesigning, and retranscribing.

# 15

# Active Reach

*Step 5*

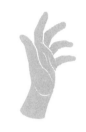

A
ctive reaches are the challenging but fun part of this plan because they are actions and exercises you say and/or do during the course of the day and evening. You in essence practice using the new healthy thought until it becomes automatized like a good habit (see chap. 8). You decide what these active reaches will be in steps 4 and 5 each day and then you monitor, evaluate, and change them each subsequent day of the 21-Day Brain Detox Plan.

## The Doing Gets the Results

It is the *doing* nature of the active reaches that results in *ungluing* the branches from your thought trees. Steps 1–4 have loosened and weakened the branches, but step 5 literally destroys the branches. Here is how this works, and why the active reaches are so important.

## Inside the Brain

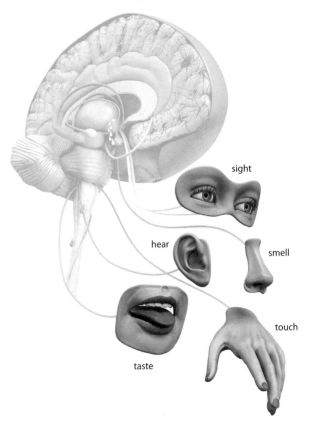

The branches with all the memories and emotions are attached to a cell body with a type of protein that is like glue—like branches attached to a tree trunk. There is more glue on the branches that are used the most, so when you shift your attention from the negative, toxic thought to the positive, healthy, new replacement thought, three things happen.

1. The electromagnetic and quantum signals from your decision to change attack the branches of the toxic

thoughts, weakening them because the signals are more powerful than the negative thoughts.

2. This causes neurochemicals to flow like oxytocin, which remolds; dopamine, which increases motivation and focus; and serotonin, which makes you feel good. These chemicals also weaken the toxic branches.

3. The "glue" starts moving away from the toxic tree to the healthy tree.

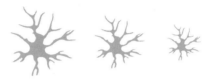

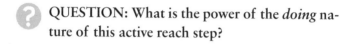

**QUESTION: What is the power of the *doing* nature of this active reach step?**

### Your Faith Manifests

The active reach is the stage in which you reach out beyond toxic thinking by applying the principle, "Faith without works is dead" (James 2:20). This is where your faith manifests and you actually do something with the detoxing that has been going on until now—you reach further. It is the final step to switching on the brain and detoxing. But you can't reach with success without the foundation created in the previous steps. Only when you have been through all of those steps and completed the process can you move forward, changed in a positive direction.

An active reach is not just the decision to forgive; it is the actual forgiving. It is not just the decision to believe that God heals; it is the actual believing. It is not just the decision to stop worrying about your children and trust they will make the right decisions because God is watching over them; it is actually stopping the worrying. It is not just confessing God will meet your needs; it is the actual believing. It is not just the decision to lose weight; it is the actual lifestyle change to lose the weight. It is not just the decision to stop dwelling on the past; it is the actual stopping the dwelling on the past. It is not just the decision not to talk negatively; it is the actual not talking negatively no matter how tempting it is to do so. This is when you reach beyond where you are.

## Moving through the Sequence

When you have moved through the 5-Step sequence—gather, reflect, write, revisit, active reach—to detox your thoughts and simultaneously build the healthy thought, you will have built a secure foundation for change, health, and wholeness. It will not work, however, if you just mouth a positive confession without a solid foundation. This creates what science calls "cognitive dissonance."

Building a structure for change on a faulty foundation will never create persistent patterns in your brain to bring you peace. Instead, it will fall down when the proverbial wolf (trouble) blows down your house of sticks (confessions without foundation).

## Integrity in the Brain

In the brain, building a foundation is called having integrity, which means you are using your words and actions to line up the thought with its beliefs and feelings. Neuroscientifically, the progression goes like this:

- the amygdala provides input to the mind about the emotions—*gather*;

- the thalamus and hypothalamus provide input on motivation; *and* the memory networks provide information on the *existing memories—reflect*;
- the central hub in the brain mixes and integrates this all together—*write*; and
- the heart acts as the checking station, and you make the decision—*revisit*.

You can be presented with all the reason, logic, scientific evidence, and just plain common sense in the world, but you won't believe something is true unless your brain's limbic system—the central location of your emotions—allows you to feel that it is true. So you can't imagine and feel—change your brain structurally—one way and speak something different, because if you do, there will be a lack of integrity operating in your brain, which will leave an overwhelming feeling of being out of control.

## Active Reaching Helps You Feel Truth

The active reach helps you feel whether or not something is true. It helps you line up the thought (imagination) with the confession (words coming out of your mouth) and action. Clearly, then, "Confess with your mouth the Lord Jesus *and* believe in your heart" (Rom. 10:9, emphasis mine) becomes the principle operating here.

Here is an example of active reach: You are working on the toxic thought of saying—out loud or in your mind—a lot of could-have, would-have, should-have, if-only statements. Your active reach step is saying, "I will not say this, I am putting the past behind me"; or visualizing the situation, event, or issue disappearing in a puff of smoke; or quoting a verse that's applicable; or doing something fun like smiling, yawning, or tapping your foot.

A second example: If the toxic thought is that you keep trying to change the past by playing movies in your mind, thinking that if you did *that* then *this* would have happened, and then *this* should have happened, and then you wouldn't have . . . active reach is to say, "I choose to stop playing this movie" or "I am switching that movie off," quoting a Bible verse that applies, or praying a prayer you have created for that situation.

A third example: The toxic thought is that you find it hard to accept that something is over, done, and in the past, and you won't let it go. The active reach is to visualize the walls of Jericho falling down and see those walls as this past experience; telling yourself "I can't" is a decision, but so is "I can"—choose "I can" or quote a Scripture.

You can't trick yourself, and you can't trick God. After all, you are made in his image and are, therefore, exceptionally intelligent. Now using your exceptional intelligence, look at the simple summary below of how to do the 21-Day Brain Detox Plan and start renewing your mind and rewiring your brain.

## Summary for the 21-Day Brain Detox Plan

1. You do the 5 steps of the Switch On Your Brain technique daily for 21 days on one specific toxic thought.

2. It takes you seven to ten minutes to work through the 5 steps, and then you do your selected active reach at least seven times throughout the day. So the active reach, step 5, has an action component that you *do* throughout the day. You have worked out what your active reach would be through using the insight you gained from steps 1–4.

3. One brain detox cycle is 21 days.

4. You can do as many 21-day cycles as you need on the same toxic thought to rewire it, but most times one cycle will do.

5. You are simultaneously breaking down a toxic thought and building up a healthy thought.

6. You need to practice automatizing the new healthy tree by consciously practicing using it for at least two more 21-day cycles.

Below is a guide to help you master the 21-Day Brain Detox.

## Learning to Break Down the Toxic Thought

1. Gather (1–2 minutes)
   - Purpose: bring thought into consciousness
   - Example: worrying about money
   - Don't forget, it is the Holy Spirit who "will guide you into all the truth" (John 16:13 NIV), so let him—and not yourself or someone else—make the decision about what you need to renew.
   - Activity: go to chapter 11 for all the step 1 gather questions to guide you.

2. Focused Reflection (1–2 minutes)
   - Purpose: loosen up branches
   - Activity: review chapter 12

3. Writing (1–2 minutes)
   - Purpose: start shaking the branches to loosen the glue
   - Activity: review chapter 13

4. Revisit (1–2 minutes)
   - Purpose: shift the glue to the new healthy thought
   - Activity: review chapter 14
5. Active Reach (1–2 minutes)
   - Purpose: start melting down the branches
   - Activity: review chapter 15

## Learning to Build Up the Healthy Thought

Now let's look at the parallel building-up process, which you do at exactly the same time as you do the breaking-down process to balance the negative with the positive. You don't want to get stuck in the negative—toxicity—so you immediately bring balance to the situation.

1. **Gather**
   - As you identify the toxic thought in the breaking-down process, you immediately, prayerfully, consciously think of the replacement thought. For example: "My God will supply every need of yours according to his riches in glory in Christ Jesus" (Phil. 4:19 ESV). (See chap. 11.)
2. **Focused Reflection**
   - Grow and integrate healthy branches by reflecting on the positive and not just dwelling on the negative. (See chap. 12.)
3. **Write**
   - Add more information and links with other branches by writing the positive alongside the negative. (See chap. 13.)
4. **Revisit**
   - You are doing the same thing in the breaking-down and building-up processes here. The steps cross over

because you are planning the solution to replace the problem. This starts stabilizing the branches to firm up the "glue" bonds. (See chap. 14.)

5. **Active Reach**

- This is the same step as in the breaking-down process, but here you actually *do* the active reaches. This strengthens the new thought branches. (See chap. 15.)

Repeating steps 1 through 5 daily for about seven minutes eventually eliminates the toxic tree and stabilizes the healthy tree. Like the Scripture says in Mark 11:22–23, "You can say to this mountain, 'May you be lifted up and thrown into the sea,' and it will happen" (NLT).

# Afterword

As I sat down to write this, I wondered why it is that certain things stick in your brain. Then I thought, *Why is it that the guy writing an afterword for a book about how the brain works is asking questions about how the brain works? Why don't I just read the book and get my answers?* Caroline certainly answers my enigma in these pages.

Let me digress. For me, some of the "stuck" memories are events, locations, smells, feelings, visions, and dreams. Some are good; some are not as good. Diesel exhaust is a real bummer of a memory for me; it can almost immediately make me nauseated. (I went to Israel numerous times as a teenager, and traveled the length and breadth of the Holy Land by diesel-belching buses.) When I feel extreme cold, I think of football. (I opened the door of a hotel one time in Detroit for Lions' great Hall of Famer Barry Sanders.)

The geometry definition "two lines cut by a transversal so that alternate interior angles are congruent and the lines are parallel" is burnt into my brain. (I was rudely awakened

203

from an awesome daydream and then traumatized by a math teacher summoning me to the blackboard to solve a math equation from another planet in front of my entire class.)

When Laurie, my wife of almost thirty years now, tilts her head at a certain angle to look up at me, I feel a "slap a ring on that girl's finger and run down the aisle and get married" kind of LOVE. I am taken back to the fall of 1984, standing in Pastor Don Price's church embracing her, instantly in love, holding her longer, tighter, and wondering how many people were like, *Um . . . What's up with the major PDA in church!* We were hardly ever apart after that fateful evening and married a few months later.

When I am introduced to a person named Tom and/or sometimes just hear the name Tom, I want to giggle, seriously! My brain can replay a movie of Laurie looking at but past me, eyes going wide like she was seeing a ghost over my shoulder! (We were at a friend's home in Los Angeles for a dinner party, and unbeknownst to me two-time Academy award–winning actor Tom Hanks was standing behind me, waiting to say hello to our host, but I was mid-story and rambling on and on, and Laurie was desperately trying to tell me to shut up and turn around with her "Lucy Ricardo" eye gestures! I finally did, and Tom said, "Hi, I'm Tom." I said, "Yes, I know.")

When I see an advertisement for a certain global technology company that manufactures telephone systems, tears can well up in my eyes. I answered a phone call in 1991 to the sounds of sobbing on the other end of the line. (Laurie choked out the news to me that she had miscarried our second child.) I can remember where I was when I heard about President Reagan being shot; the Challenger disaster; September 11, 2001; the birth of my boys, Caylan and Cody, their first steps, birthday cake being smashed into faces, etc.

Hopefully you are tracking with me here. I pray you are able to conjure up your own random memories, good and not so good, and are asking the same questions I am. Why do these events become us, become the very persona of who we are? Why *those* memories? What makes them "stick" in our brains?

This book is the owner's manual for how our brain works. Refer to it regularly. Caroline Leaf's first appearance on TBN's *Praise The Lord* program with Laurie and me is one of the "stuck" memories in my brain too. I remember thinking that I was not listening to a doctor's opinion regarding how God created our brains but was actually hearing a revelation that was divinely inspired. I vividly recall saying, "Let me repeat what I think you just said. Our thoughts are actually 'proteins' forming the way our brains will actually think about matters in the future? So the Scripture that says, 'as a man thinks, so is he' actually means that 'as a man thinks, so is he'? Wow! Science is actually catching up with the Bible!"

That was Caroline's first program with us. She has taught us more and more truth over the years, and is now in production on an entire TV series that will air on TBN for years!

These pages are not information—they are revelation. And Caroline's revelation will change the way you think.

Literally!

Matthew Crouch,
Trinity Broadcasting Family of Networks

# Notes

## Chapter 1 Mind Controls Matter

1. Eric R. Kandel, *In Search of Memory: The Emergence of a New Science of Mind* (New York: Norton, 2006).

2. Sigmund Freud, quoted in D. Church, *The Genie in Your Genes* (Fulton, CA: Energy Psychology Press, 2008).

3. Norman Doidge, *The Brain That Changes Itself: Stories of Personal Triumph from the Frontiers of Brain Science* (New York: Penguin Books, 2007); Joe Dispenza, *Evolve Your Brain: The Science of Changing Your Brain* (Deerfield Beach, FL: Health Communications, 2007); Henry Markram, director of the Brain and Mind Institute of the *Ecole Polytechnique Fédérale de Lausanne* that founded the Blue Brain Project, which accurately predicts connections between neurons, *Science Daily*, September 17, 2012, www.sciencedaily.com /releases/2012/09/120917152043.htm?utm_source=feedburner&utm_medium=email&utm_campaign=Feed%3A+sciencedaily%2Fmind_brain%2Fneuro science+%28ScienceDaily%3A+Mind+%26+Brain+News+—+Neuroscience%29; and Allan Jones, http://www.ted.com/speakers/allan_jones.html.

4. 98 percent of mental and physical illnesses come from our thought life: www.stress.org/americas.htm; www.naturalwellnesscare.com/stress-statistics.html; Harvard Medical School's Mind-Body Institute, www.massgeneral.org/bhi/research/; Church, *Genie in Your Genes*. The Institute of HeartMath discusses an experiment titled "Local and Nonlocal Effects of Coherent Heart Frequencies on Conformational Changes of DNA." http://appreciativeinquiry.case.edu/practice/organizationDetail.cfm?coid=852&sector=21. A study by the American Medical Association found that stress is a factor in 75 percent of all illnesses and diseases that people suffer from today. The association between stress and disease is a colossal 85 percent, Brian Luke Seaward, www.brianlukeseaward.net/articles/SuperStress-WELCOA-Seaward.pdf.

"Cancer Statistics and Views of Causes," *Science News* 115, no. 2 (January 13, 1979): 23; H. F. Nijhout "Metaphors and the Role of Genes and Development," *BioEssays* 12 (1990): 444–46; W. C. Willett, "Balancing Lifestyle and Genomics Research for Disease

Prevention," *Science* 296 (2002): 695–98; C. B. Pert, *Molecules of Emotion: Why You Feel the Way You Feel* (New York: Simon and Schuster, 1997); B. Lipton, *The Biology of Belief: Unleashing the Power of Consciousness, Matter and Miracles* (Santa Cruz, CA: Mountain of Love Productions, 2008).

    5. C. M. Leaf, *The Gift in You: Discover New Life through Gifts Hidden in Your Mind* (Nashville: Thomas Nelson, 2009).

    6. Church, *Genie in Your Genes.*

    7. Herbert Benson MD, president of Harvard Medical School's Mind-Body Institute, www.massgeneral.org/bhi/research.

    8. Glen Rein and Rollin McCraty, "Local and Nonlocal Effects of Coherent Heart Frequencies on Conformational Changes of DNA," Proceedings of the Joint USPA/IAPR Psychotronics Conference, Milwaukee, Wisconsin, 1993, http://www.heartmath.org/templates/ihm/e-newsletter/publication/2012/winter/emotions-can-change-your-dna.php; Rollin McCraty et al., "Modulation of DNA Conformation By Heart-focused Intention." HeartMath Research Center, Institute of HeartMath, publications no. 03–08, Boulder Creek, CA, 2003.

    9. "Stress," Your Dictionary, http://www.yourdictionary.com/stress. Emphasis mine.

    10. Sheldon Cohen et al., "Psychological Stress and Disease," *JAMA* 14 (2007): 1685, http://www.bbc.com/future/story/20120619-how-stress-could-cause-illness; http://www.stress.org/stress-and-heart-disease/.

    11. Brian Luke Seaward, *Managing Stress: Principles and Strategies for Health and Wellbeing* (London: Jones and Bartlett Learning, 2006).

    12. "Cancer Statistics and Views of Causes," *Science News* 115, no. 2 (January 13, 1979): 23.

    13. Lipton, *The Biology of Belief.*

    14. Nijhout, "Metaphors and the Role of Genes and Development."

    15. Willett, "Balancing Lifestyle and Genomics Research for Disease Prevention."

    16. "Stress and Heart Disease," http://www.stress.org/stress-and-heart-disease/.

## Chapter 2 Choice and Your Multiple-Perspective Advantage

    1. Jeffery Rosen, "The Brain on the Stand," *New York Times*, March 11, 2007, www.nytimes.com/2007/03/11/magazine/11Neurolaw.t.html.

    2. Francis Crick, quoted in John Tierney, "Do You Have Free Will? Yes, It's the Only Choice," *New York Times*, March 21, 2011, www.nytimes.com/2011/03/22/science/22tier.html?pagewanted=all&_r=0.

    3. Benjamin Libet, "Unconscious Cerebral Initiative and the Role of Conscious Will in Voluntary Action," *Behavioral and Brain Sciences* 8 (1985): 529–66; John Dylan-Haynes et al., "Unconscious Determinants of Free Decisions in the Human Brain," *Nature Neuroscience* 11 (2008): 543–45.

    4. Hagop Sarkissian et al., "Is Belief in Free Will a Cultural Universal?" *Mind and Language* 25 (2010): 346–58.

    5. Kathleen D. Vohs and Jonathan W. Schooler, "The Value of Believing in Free Will: Encouraging a Belief in Determinism Increases Cheating," www.csom.umn.edu/assets/91974.pdf.

    6. Articles in *Science* and *NewScientist* have recently discussed x-phi work on free will from authors including Eddy Nahmias and Dylan Murray, "Experimental Philosophy on Free Will: An Error Theory for Incompatibilist Intuitions," in *New Waves in Philosophy of Action*, ed. Jess Aguilar, Andrei Buckareff, and Keith Frankish (Basingstoke,

Hampshire, UK: Palgrave-Macmillan, 2011); and Eddy Nahmias, Stephen G. Morris, Thomas Nadelhoffer, and Jason Turner "Is Incompatibilism Intuitive?" *Philosophy and Phenomenological Research* 73, no. 1 (2006): 28–53.

7. H. S. Mayberg, "Defining the Neural Circuitry of Depression: Toward a New Nosology with Therapeutic Implications," *Biological Psychiatry* 61, no. 6 (March 2007): 729–30.

8. Church, *Genie in Your Genes*; "Epigenetics: A Web Tour," *Science*, www.sciencemag. org/feature/plus/sfg/resources/res_epigenetics.dtl.; Ethan Watters, "DNA Is Not Destiny: The New Science of Epigenetics Rewrites the Rules of Disease, Heredity, and Identity," *Discover*, November 2006, http://discovermagazine.com/2006/nov/cover.

9. Elizabeth Pennisi, "Behind the Scenes of Gene Expression," *Science* 293, no. 553 (2001): 1064–67.

10. Ibid.

11. Ken Richardson, *The Making of Intelligence* (New York: Columbia University Press, 2000).

12. Eric R. Kandel, James H. Schwartz, and Thomas M. Jessell, eds. *Essentials of Neural Science and Behavior* (New York: Appleton and Lange, 1995); Eric R. Kandel, "Molecular Biology of Memory: A Dialogue between Genes and Synapses," http://www. nobelprize.org/mediaplayer/index.php?id=1447; Eric. R. Kandel, "A New Intellectual Framework for Psychiatry," *American Journal of Psychiatry* 155, no. 4 (1998): 457–69.

13. Ibid.

14. Dorothy Nelkin, *The DNA Mystique* (New York: Norton, 1995), 15.

15. Lipton, *Biology of Belief*. B. Lipton, K. G. Bensch, and M. A. Karasek, "Microvessel Endothelial Cell Transdifferentiation: Phenotypic Characterization," *Differentiation* 46 (1991): 117–33.

16. Gail Ironson et al., "An Increase in Religiousness/Spirituality Occurs after HIV Diagnosis and Predicts Slower Disease Progression over Four Years in People with HIV," *Journal of General Internal Medicine* 21 (2006): 62–68.

17. As quoted in Church, *Genie in Your Genes*, 65.

## Chapter 3 Your Choices Change Your Brain

1. Watters, "DNA Is Not Destiny."

2. John Cloud, "Why Your DNA Isn't Your Destiny," *Time*, www.time.com/time/magazine/article/0,9171,1952313-2,00.html.

3. Robert Weinhold, "Epigenetics: The Science of Change," *Environmental Health Perspectives* 114, no. 3 (March 2006).

4. "Learning Without Learning," *The Economist*, September 21, 2006, 89.

5. www.cajal.csic.es/ingles/index.html.

6. In part 2, I will explain how this can be done.

7. Jeffrey M. Schwartz and Sharon Begley, *The Mind and the Brain* (New York: Harper Perennial, 2002); Jeffrey M. Schwartz and Rebecca Gladding, *You Are Not Your Brain* (New York: Avery, 2012).

8. Caroline M. Leaf, "The Mind Mapping Approach: A Model and Framework for Geodesic Learning" (unpublished doctoral dissertation, University of Pretoria, Pretoria, South Africa, 1997); Caroline M. Leaf, Brenda Louw, and Isabel Uys, "The Development of a Model for Geodesic Learning: The Geodesic Information Processing Model," *The South African Journal of Communication Disorders* 44 (1997): 53–70; Leaf, "The Move from Institution Based Rehabilitation (IBR) to Community Based

Rehabilitation (CBR): A Paradigm Shift," *Therapy Africa* 1, no. 1 (August 1997): 4; Leaf, "An Altered Perception of Learning: Geodesic Learning," *Therapy Africa* 1, no. 2 (October 1997): 7.

9. Doidge, *Brain That Changes Itself*.

10. Barbara Arrowsmith and Norman Doidge, *The Woman Who Changed Her Brain: And Other Inspiring Stories of Pioneering Brain Transformation* (New York: Free Press, 2012).

11. Caroline M. Leaf, *The Switch On Your Brain 5-Step Learning Process* (Dallas: Switch On Your Brain, 2008).

12. Arrowsmith and Doidge, *Woman Who Changed Her Brain*; Church, *Genie in Your Genes*; Doidge, *Brain That Changes Itself*; Dispenza, *Evolve Your Brain*; Leaf, "Mind Mapping Approach"; Leaf, *Switch On Your Brain 5-Step Learning Process*; Caroline M. Leaf, *Who Switched Off My Brain? Controlling Toxic Thoughts and Emotions* (Dallas: Switch on Your Brain, 2007) and DVD series (Johannesburg, South Africa: Switch on Your Brain, 2007); C. M. Leaf, M. Copeland, and J. Maccaro, "Your Body His Temple: God's Plan for Achieving Emotional Wholeness," DVD series (Dallas: Life Outreach International, 2007).

13. Joe Dispenza, *Breaking the Habit of Being Yourself* (New York: Hay House, 2012).

14. Richard Wiseman, "Self Help: Forget Positive Thinking, Try Positive Action," *The Observer*, June 30, 2012, http://www.guardian.co.uk/science/2012/jun/30/self-help-positive-thinking; Jim Taylor, "Is the Self-help Industry a Fraud?" April 18, 2011, http://blog.ctnews.com/taylor/2011/04/18/is-the-self-help-industry-a-fraud/#.UVedEdRXVA4. email; Michael Shermer, "SHAM Scam: The Self-Help and Actualization Movement Has Become an $8.5-Billion-a-Year Business. Does It Work?" April 23, 2006, http://www.scientificamerican.com/article.cfm?id=sham-scam.

15. "The Problem with Self-Help Books: Study Shows the Negative Side to Positive Self-Statements," *e! Science News*, July 2, 2009, http://esciencenews.com/articles/2009/07/02/the.problem.with.self.help.books.study.shows.negative.side.positive.self.statements.

16. Schwartz and Begley, *Mind and the Brain*; Schwartz and Gladding, *You Are Not Your Brain*.

## Chapter 4 Catch Those Thoughts

1. Ellen Langer and Mihnea Moldoveanu, "The Construct of Mindfulness," *Journal of Social Issues* 56, no. 1 (2000): 1–9; Leaf, *Who Switched Off My Brain?*; Leaf, *The Gift in You*.

2. Caroline M. Leaf, Isabel C. Uys, and Brenda Louw, "An Alternative Non-Traditional Approach to Learning: The Metacognitive-Mapping Approach." *The South African Journal of Communication Disorders* 45 (1998): 87–102.

3. Sissa Medialab, "The Good Side of the Prion: A Molecule That Is Not Only Dangerous, but Can Help the Brain Grow," *Science Daily*, February 14, 2013, www.sciencedaily.com/releases/2013/02/130214075437.htm?utm_source=feedburner&utm_medium=email&utm_campaign=Feed%3A+sciencedaily%2Fmind_brain+%28Science Daily%3A+Mind+%26+Brain+News%29.

4. Loyola University Health System, "New Evidence for Link between Depression and Heart Disease," *Science Daily*, February 18, 2013.

5. "Brain Signs of Schizophrenia Found in Babies," *Science Daily*, June 9, 2010, http://www.sciencedaily.com/releases/2010/06/100621111240.htm; "Alterations in Brain

Activity in Children at Risk of Schizophrenia Predate Onset of Symptoms," *Science Daily*, March 22, 2013, http://www.sciencedaily.com/releases/2013/03/130322174343.htm.

6. Leaf, *Who Switched Off My Brain?*; Maria Konnikova, *Mastermind: How to Think Like Sherlock Holmes* (New York: Viking Penguin, 2013); Maria Konnikova, "The Power of Concentration," *New York Times Sunday Review*, December 15, 2012, http://www.nytimes.com/2012/12/16/opinion/sunday/the-power-of-concentration.html ?pagewanted=1&_r=2&ref=general&src=me&.

7. Schwartz and Begley, *Mind and the Brain*; Schwartz and Gladding, *You Are Not Your Brain*; Dispenza, *Evolve Your Brain*; Dispenza, *Breaking the Habit of Being Yourself*; Allan Jones, www.ted.com/speakers/allan_jones.html.

## Chapter 5 Entering into Directed Rest

1. Richard J. Davidson et al., "Alterations in Brain and Immune Function Produced by Mindfulness Meditation," *Psychosomatic Medicine* 65 (2003): 564–70.

2. Marcus E. Raichle et al., "A Default Mode of Brain Function: A Brief History of an Evolving Idea," *Neuroimage* 37 (2007): 1083–90.

3. Matthew R. Brier et al., "Loss of Intranetwork and Internetwork Resting State Functional Connections with Alzheimer's Disease Progression," *Journal of Neuroscience* 32, no. 26 (2012): 8890–99; Christian F. Beckmann et al., "Investigations into Resting-State Connectivity Using Independent Component Analysis," *Philos Trans R Soc Lond, B, Biol Sci* 360 (2005):1001–13.

4. Marcus E. Raichle, "The Brain's Dark Energy," *Scientific American*, March 20, 2012, 44–49, www.hboorcca.com/pdf/brain/The%20Brain's%20Dark%20Energy%20 Scientific%20American%20March%202010.pdf; Raichle et al., "A Default Mode of Brain Function," 1083–90.

5. Yvette I. Sheline et al., "The Default Mode Network and Self-Referential Processes in Depression," *Proceedings of the National Academy of Sciences USA* 106, no. 6 (January 26, 2009): 1942–47; Washington University School of Medicine research cited in "Alzheimer's Breaks Brain Networks' Coordination," *Science Daily*, September 17, 2012, www.sciencedaily.com/releases/2012/09/120918090812.htm.

6. Raichle, "The Brain's Dark Energy"; Raichle et al., "A Default Mode of Brain Function."

7. Konnikova, "The Power of Concentration."

8. Brier et al., "Loss of Intranetwork and Internetwork Resting State Functional Connections with Alzheimer's Disease Progression."

9. J. Paul Hamilton et al., "Default Mode and Task Positive Network Activity in Major Depressive Disorder: Implications for Adaptive and Maladaptive Rumination," *Biological Psychiatry* 70, no. 4 (2011): 327–33.

10. Caroline M. Leaf, "Mind Mapping: A Therapeutic Technique for Closed Head Injury," unpublished master's dissertation (University of Pretoria, Pretoria, South Africa), 1990.

11. "Activity in Brain Networks Related to Features of Depression," *Science Daily*, April 3, 2012, www.sciencedaily.com/releases/2012/04/120403111954.htm#.T4HbzA jE61c.mailto.

12. Xueling Zhu et al., "Evidence of a Dissociation Pattern in Resting-State Default Mode Network Connectivity in First-Episode, Treatment-Naive Major Depression Patients," *Biological Psychiatry* 71, no. 7 (2012): 611.

13. Norman A. S. Farb et al., "Mood-Linked Responses in Medial Prefrontal Cortex Predict Relapse in Patients with Recurrent Unipolar Depression," *Biological Psychiatry* 70, no. 4 (August 15, 2011): 366–72.

14. Leaf, "The Mind Mapping Approach"; Hamilton et al., "Default Mode and Task Positive Network Activity in Major Depressive Disorder."

15. Sophie Green et al., "Guilt-Selective Functional Disconnection of Anterior Temporal and Subgenual Cortices in Major Depressive Disorder," *Archives of General Psychiatry* 69, no. 10 (2012): 1014–21, http://archpsyc.jamanetwork.com/article.aspx?articleID=1171078.

16. Ibid.

17. Schwartz and Begley, *Mind and the Brain*; Schwartz and Gladding, *You Are Not Your Brain*.

18. Michael M. Merzenich et al., "Prophylactic Reduction and Remediation of Schizophrenic Impairments through Interactive Behavioral Training," 2001, http://www.google.com/patents?hl=en&lr=&vid=USPAT6231344&id=3BQIAAAAEBAJ&oi=fnd&dq=Merzenich+schizophrenia+research&printsec=abstract#v=onepage&q=Merzenich%20schizophrenia%20research&f=false; Melissa Fisher et al., "Neuroplasticity-Based Cognitive Training in Schizophrenia: An Interim Report on the Effects 6 Months Later," *Schizophrenia Bulletin*, March 5, 2009, http://schizophreniabulletin.oxfordjournals.org/content/36/4/869; "Thread: New Therapy Available Now for Cognitive problems in Schizophrenia," http://www.schizophrenia.com:8080/jiveforums/thread.jspa?threadID=16719; Sophia Vinogradov, "What's New in Schizophrenia Research," November 28, 2007, http://www.thomastthomas.com/Schizophrenia%20Research,Vinogradov,112807.pdf.

19. Sarah J. Hart et al., "Altered fronto-limbic activity in children and adolescents with familial high risk for schizophrenia," *Psychiatry Research* 212, no. 1 (2013): 19; Sebastien Parnaudeau et al., "Inhibition of Mediodorsal Thalamus Disrupts Thalamofrontal Connectivity and Cognition," *Neuron* 77, no. 6 (2013): 1151.

20. "Women Abused as Children More Likely to Have Children With Autism," *Science Daily*, March 20, 2013, http://www.sciencedaily.com/releases/2013/03/130320212818.htm#.UVCuOUPuaJE.email.

## Chapter 6  Stop Milkshake-Multitasking

1. Brian A. Primack et al., "Association Between Media Use in Adolescence and Depression in Young Adulthood," *Archives of General Psychiatry* 66, no. 2 (2009): 181–88, http://archpsyc.jamanetwork.com/article.aspx?articleid=210196.

2. Mark W. Becker, Reem Alzahabi, and Christopher J. Hopwood, "Media Multitasking Is Associated with Symptoms of Depression and Social Anxiety," *Cyberpsychology, Behavior, and Social Networking* 16, no. 2 (2012): 132–35.

3. "Are You a Facebook Addict?" *Science Daily*, May 7, 2012, www.sciencedaily.com/releases/2012/05/120507102054.htm.

4. Report from the University of Edinburgh Business School, "More Facebook Friends Means More Stress, Says Report," *Science Daily*, November 26, 2012, www.sciencedaily.com/releases/2012/11/121126131218.htm.

5. Keith Wilcox and Andrew T. Stephen, "Are Close Friends the Enemy? Online Social Networks, Self-Esteem, and Self-Control," *Social Science Research Network*, September 22, 2012, http://ssrn.com/abstract=2155864.

6. David M. Levy et al., "The Effects of Mindfulness Meditation Training on Multitasking in a High-Stress Information Environment," *Proceedings of Graphics Interface*, May 2012; University of Washington research referenced in "Mindful Multitasking: Meditation First Can Calm Stress, Aid Concentration," *Science Daily*, June 13, 2012, www.sciencedaily.com/releases/2012/06/120614094118.htm.

7. Leaf, "Mind Mapping: A Therapeutic Technique for Closed Head Injury"; Leaf, "The Mind Mapping Approach."

8. University of Washington study cited in Konnikova, "The Power of Concentration."

9. University of Washington and Emory University studies referenced in Konnikova, "The Power of Concentration"; Michael Merzenich, cited in Schwartz and Begley, *Mind and the Brain*; Gaëlle Desbordes et al., "Effects of Mindful-Attention and Compassion Meditation Training on Amygdala Response to Emotional Stimuli in an Ordinary, Non-Meditative State," *Frontiers in Human Neuroscience*, November 1, 2012, www.frontiersin.org/human_neuroscience/10.3389/fnhum.2012.00292/abstract.

10. Michael Merzenich cited in Schwartz and Begley, *Mind and the Brain*. Desbordes et al., "Effects of Mindful-Attention and Compassion Meditation Training on Amygdala Response to Emotional Stimuli in an Ordinary, Non-Meditative State"; Massachusetts General Hospital, Boston University, "Meditation Appears to Produce Enduring Changes in Emotional Processing in the Brain," *Science Daily*, www.sciencedaily.com/releases/2012/11/121112150339.htm.

11. Leaf, "Mind Mapping: A Therapeutic Technique for Closed Head Injury."

12. Eileen Luders et al., "The Unique Brain Anatomy of Meditation Practitioners: Alterations in Cortical Gyrification," *Frontiers in Human Neuroscience*, February 29, 2012, www.frontiersin.org/Human_Neuroscience/10.3389/fnhum.2012.00034/abstract.

13. Eileen Luders et al., "Enhanced Brain Connectivity in Long-Term Meditation Practitioners," *NeuroImage* 4 (August 15, 2011): 1308–16.

14. University of California, Los Angeles research cited in "Meditation May Increase Gray Matter," *Science Daily*, May 13, 2009, www.sciencedaily.com/releases/2009/05/090512134655.htm.

## Chapter 7 Thinking, God, and the Quantum Physics Brain

1. "Max Planck Quotes," www.goodreads.com/author/quotes/107032.Max_Planck.

2. Schwartz and Begley, *Mind and the Brain*; Schwartz and Gladding, *You Are Not Your Brain*; Jeffrey Schwartz, Henry Stapp, and Mario Beauregard, "Quantum Physics in Neuroscience and Psychology: A Neurophysical Model of Mind/Brain Interaction," www.physics.lbl.gov/~stapp/PTB6.pdf.

3. This intentional mental act and its unpredictability can be represented mathematically by an equation that is one of the key components of quantum theory. It is beyond the scope of this book to explore the equation more deeply, but if you are interested, you can begin exploring further by reading, "Quantum Physics in Neuroscience and Psychology: A Neurophysical Model of Mind/Brain Interaction," by Jeffrey M. Schwartz, Henry P. Stapp, and Mario Beauregard, http://www.scribd.com/doc/94124369/Quantum-Physics-in-Neuroscience-by-Jeffrey-M-Schwartz-Henry-P-Stapp-Mario-Beauregard.

4. James Higgo, "A Lazy Layman's Guide to Quantum Physics," 1999, www.higgo.com/quantum/laymans.htm.

5. Schwartz, Stapp, and Beauregard, "Quantum Physics in Neuroscience and Psychology."

6. Schwartz and Begley, *Mind and the Brain*; Schwartz and Gladding, *You Are Not Your Brain*; Schwartz, Stapp, and Beauregard, "Quantum Physics in Neuroscience and Psychology."

7. Caroline Leaf, "The Mind Mapping Approach: A Model and Framework for Geodesic Learning," unpublished DPhil dissertation, University of Pretoria, South Africa, 1997; Caroline Leaf, "The Mind Mapping Approach: A Technique for Closed Head Injury," unpublished master's dissertation, University of Pretoria, South Africa, 1990.

8. Carol Dweck, "Implicit Theories of Intelligence Predict Achievement Across Adolescent Transition: A Longitudinal Study and an Intervention," *Child Development* 78 (2007): 246–63.

9. McCraty, "Modulation of DNA Conformation by Heart-Focused Intention," 4.

10. Church, *Genie in Your Genes*.

11. Giacomo Rizzolatti and L. Craighero, "The Mirror-Neuron System," *Annual Review of Neuroscience* 27 (2004): 169–92.

12. Caroline Leaf, *Who Switched Off Your Brain? Solving the Mystery of He Said/ She Said* (Nashville: Thomas Nelson, 2011).

13. Dean Radin, "Testing Nonlocal Observation as a Source of Intuitive Knowledge," *Explore* 4, no. 1 (2008): 25.

14. Thomas E. Oxman et al., "Lack of Social Participation or Religious Strength and Comfort as Risk Factors for Death after Cardiac Surgery in the Elderly," *Psychosomatic Medicine* 57 (1995): 5.

15. Linda H. Powell et al., "Religion and Spirituality: Linkages to Physical Health," *American Psychologist* 58, no. 1 (2003): 36.

16. Larry Dossey, *Prayer Is Good Medicine* (San Francisco: HarperOne, 1997).

17. John A. Astin et al., "The Efficacy of 'Distant Healing': A Systematic Review of Randomized Trials," *Annals of Internal Medicine* 12 (2000): 903; Wayne B. Jonas, "The Middle Way: Realistic Randomized Controlled Trials for the Evaluation of Spiritual Healing," *The Journal of Alternative and Complementary Medicine* 7, no. 1 (2001): 5–7.

18. David Levy and Joel Kilpatrick, *Gray Matter: A Neurosurgeon Discovers the Power of Prayer . . . One Patient at a Time* (Wheaton, IL: Tyndale, 2012); Matt Donnelly, "Faith Boosts Cognitive Management of HIV and Cancer," *Science & Theology News* (2006): 16.

19. Levy and Kilpatrick, *Gray Matter*, 19.

20. Sundance Bilson-Thompson, Fotini Markopoulou, and Lee Smolin, "Quantum Gravity and the Standard Model," *Classical and Quantum Gravity* 24, no. 16 (2007): 3975–93.

21. Don Lincoln, "The Universe Is a Complex and Intricate Place," *Scientific American*, November 2012, 38–43.

22. This is the terminology of the Heisenberg principle—quantum physics is known for its weird wording and almost ambiguous statements.

23. Henry Stapp, "Philosophy of Mind and the Problem of Free Will in the Light of Quantum Mechanics," www-physics.lbl.gov/~stapp/Philosophy.pdf; Henry Stapp, *Mindful Universe: Quantum Mechanics and the Participating Observer* (London: Springer, 2007).

24. Don Lincoln, "The Inner Life of Quarks," *Scientific American*, November 2012, 38.

## Chapter 8 The Science of Thought

1. Leaf, "Mind Mapping"; Leaf, "Mind Mapping Approach"; Leaf, Louw, and Uys, "Development of a Model for Geodesic Learning," 44, 53–70.

2. Thomas More, *Utopia*, updated edition (London: Penguin Classics, 2003), 81.

3. Leaf, *Switch On Your Brain 5-Step Learning Process*; Leaf, *Who Switched Off My Brain?*; Caroline M. Leaf, "Who Switched Off My Brain? Controlling Toxic Thoughts and Emotions," DVD series (Johannesburg, South Africa: Switch On Your Brain, 2007).

4. Schwartz and Begley, *Mind and the Brain*.

5. Andrew Newberg, Eugene D'Aquili, and Vince Rause, *Why God Won't Go Away: Brain Science and the Biology of Belief* (New York: Ballantine, 2001).

6. Schwartz and Begley, *Mind and the Brain*; Schwartz and Gladding, *You Are Not Your Brain*; Schwartz, Stapp, and Beauregard, "Quantum Physics in Neuroscience and Psychology."

7. Leaf, "Mind Mapping"; Leaf, "The Mind Mapping Approach"; Leaf, Louw, and Uys, "Development of a Model for Geodesic Learning," 44, 53–70.

8. Ibid.

9. "Blue Brain Project Accurately Predicts Connections between Neurons," *Science Daily*, September 17, 2012, www.sciencedaily.com/releases/2012/09/120917152043.htm.

## Chapter 9  What Is the 21-Day Brain Detox Plan?

1. Leaf, "Mind Mapping"; Leaf, "The Mind Mapping Approach"; Leaf, Louw, and Uys, "Development of a Model for Geodesic Learning," 44, 53–70.

2. Leaf, "Mind Mapping Approach: Technique for Closed Head Injury."

3. Karim Nader, http://blogs.mcgill.ca/science/2009/04/30/karim-nader-on-memory -reconsolidation; Karim Nader, Glenn E. Schafe, and Joseph E. Le Doux, "Fear Memories Require Protein Synthesis in the Amygdala for Reconsolidation after Retrieval," *Nature* 406, no. 6797 (2000): 722–26; A. H. Maslow, *Motivation and Personality* (New York: Harper & Row, 1970).

4. Shawn Achor, *The Happiness Advantage* (New York: Crown Business, 2010).

5. *Harvard Crimson* poll, 2004, cited in ibid.

## Chapter 10  How and Why the 21-Day Brain Detox Plan Works

1. This is 365 days in a year divided by 21 days in a cycle, which gives you 17 cycles per year.

2. Kandel, *In Search of Memory*.

3. Church, *Genie in Your Genes*.

4. Ibid.

5. Rodolfo Llinas, "Rodolfo Llinas's Fearless Approach to Neurophysiology Has Redefined Our Thinking about Individual Neurons and How They Create Movement and Consciousness," U. S. Columbian Medical Association, http://uscma.org/2010/09/12/ rodolfo-llinas's-fearless-approach-to-neurophysiology-has-redefined-our-thinking- about-individual-neurons-and-how-they-create-movement-and-consciousness; Rodolfo Llinas, *I of the Vortex* (Cambridge, MA: MIT Press, 2002).

6. Michael Merzenich as cited in Doidge, *Brain That Changes Itself*.

7. Phillippa Lally et al., "How Are Habits Formed: Modelling Habit Formation in the Real World," *European Journal of Social Psychology* 40, no. 6 (2010): 998–1009.

8. Ibid.

9. See K. Anders Ericsson, Michael J. Prietula, and Edward T. Cokely, "The Making of an Expert," *Harvard Business Review*, July 2007, http://hbr.org/2007/07/the -making-of-an-expert/ar/1.

## Chapter 11 Gather

1. Jennifer Wiley and Andrew F. Jarosz, "Working Memory Capacity, Attentional Focus, and Problem Solving," *Current Directions in Psychological Science* 21, no. 4 (2012): 258. See also, "Greater Working Memory Benefits Analytic, Not Creative, Problem-Solving," *Science Daily*, August 7, 2012, www.sciencedaily.com/releases/2012/08/120807132209.htm.

## Chapter 12 Focused Reflection

1. "Mindfulness Meditation May Relieve Chronic Inflammation," *Science Daily*, January 16, 2013, http://www.sciencedaily.com/releases/2013/01/130116163536.htm.

2. "Evidence Supports Health Benefits of 'Mindfulness-Based Practices,'" *Science Daily*, July 11, 2012, http://www.sciencedaily.com/releases/2012/07/120711104811.htm.

3. "Breast Cancer Survivors Benefit from Practicing Mindfulness-Based Stress Reduction," *Science Daily*, December 29, 2011, http://www.sciencedaily.com/releases/2011/12/111229203000.htm.

4. "Don't Worry, Be Happy: Understanding Mindfulness Meditation," *Science Daily*, November 1, 2011, http://www.sciencedaily.com/releases/2011/10/111031154134.htm.

5. "Mindfulness Meditation Training Changes Brain Structure in Eight Weeks," *Science Daily*, January 21, 2011, http://www.sciencedaily.com/releases/2011/01/110121144007.htm.

6. I explain this in depth in chapter 5 (key 5) and chapter 6 (key 6). It's worth taking the time to look back at these chapters at this point.

## Chapter 13 Write

1. Caroline Leaf, *The Switch On Your Brain 5-Step Learning Process DVD/Workbook* (Dallas: Switch On Your Brain, 2009).

# Recommended Reading

The concepts I teach in this book cover a wide spectrum, including years of reading, research, and working with clients in private practice as well as in schools and business corporations. If I had to provide all the citations to document the origin of each fact for complete scientific scholarship that I have used, there would be almost as many citations as words. So I have used a little more flexibility to write this book in a more popular style that communicates my message as effectively as possible. There are only a few citations in the actual text that are more general, and the book list that follows is a list of recommended reading of some of the great books and scientific articles I have used in my research.

Achor, S. *The Happiness Advantage*. New York: Crown Business, 2010.

Adams, H. B., and B. Wallace. "A Model for Curriculum Development: TASC." *Gifted Education International* 7 (1991): 194–213.

"Aging Brains Lose Less than Thought." *Harvard University Gazette*. www.news. harvard.edu/gazette/1996/10.03/AgingBrainsLose.html.

Alavi, A., and L. J. Hirsch. "Studies of Central Nervous System Disorders with Single Photon Emission Computed Tomography and Positron Emission

Tomography: Evolution Over the Past 2 Decades." *Seminars in Nuclear Medicine* 21, no. 1 (January 1991): 51–58.

Alesandrini, K. L. "Imagery: Eliciting Strategies and Meaningful Learning." In *Journal of Educational Psychology* 62 (1982): 526–30.

Allen D., and P. Amua-Quarshie et al. "Mental Health at Work" (White Paper). Pecan Ltd., Peckham, London, UK. 2004.

Allport, D. A. "Patterns and Actions: Cognitive Mechanisms and Content Specific." In *Cognitive Psychology: New Directions*. Edited by G. L. Claxton. London: Routledge and Kegan Paul, 1980.

Amen, D. G. *Change Your Brain, Change Your Life*. New York: Three Rivers Press, 1998.

———. *Magnificent Mind at Any Age*. New York: Harmony Books, 2008.

Amend, A. E. "Defining and Demystifying Baroque, Classic and Romantic Music." In *Journal of the Society for Accelerative Learning and Teaching* 14, no. 2 (1989): 91–112.

Amua-Quarshie, P. "Basalo-Cortical Interactions: The Role of the Basal Forebrain in Attention and Alzheimer's Disease." Unpublished master's thesis. Rutgers University, 2008.

Anastasi, M. W., and A. B. Newberg. "A Preliminary Study of the Acute Effects of Religious Ritual on Anxiety." *The Journal of Liberal and Complementary Medicine* 14, no. 2 (March 2008). www.liebertonline.com/doi/abs/10.1089/acm.2007.0675.

Anderson, J. R. *Cognitive Psychology and Its Complications*. 2nd ed. New York: Freeman, 1985.

Arnheim, R. "Visual Thinking in Education." *The Potential of Fantasy and Imagination*. Edited by A. Sheikll and J. Shaffer. New York: Brandon House, 1979, 215–25.

Arrowsmith, B., N. Doidge. *The Woman Who Changed Her Brain: And Other Inspiring Stories of Pioneering Brain Transformation*. New York: Free Press, 2012.

Atkins, R. C. *Dr. Atkins' Health Revolution*. Boston: Houghton Mifflin, 1990.

———. *Dr. Atkins' New Diet Revolution*. London: Ebury Press, 2003.

"Babies Born to Stressed Mothers More Likely to Be Bullied at School." *Science Daily*. November 14, 2012. http://www.sciencedaily.com/releases/2012/11/12 1114083821.htm?utm_source=feedburner&utm_medium=email&utm _campaign=Feed%3A+sciencedaily%2Fmind_brain+%28ScienceDaily%3A+ Mind+%26+Brain+News%29.

Bach-y-Rita, P., C. C. Collins, F. Saunders, B. White, and B. Scadden. "Vision Substitution by Tactile Image Projection." *Nature* 221, no. 5184 (1969): 963–64.

Barker, J. A. *Discovering the Future: A Question of Paradigms*. Johannesburg, South Africa: Charterhouse Productions, South African Breweries, 1987.

Bartlett, F. C. *Remembering: A Study in Experimental and Social Psychology*. Cambridge, UK: Cambridge University Press, 1932.

"Basic and Translational Neuroscience. 30th Annual Postgraduate Review Course, Topics and Speakers." December 1, 2007–March 8, 2008. http://cumc.columbia. edu/dept/cme/neuroscience/neuro/speakers.html.

Baxter, R., S. B. Cohen, and M. Ylvisaker. "Comprehensive Cognitive Assessment." *Head Injury Rehabilitation: Children and Adolescents*. Edited by M. Ylvisaker. San Diego: College-Hill Press, 1984, 247–75.

Beauregard, M., and D. O'Leary. *The Spiritual Brain*. New York: Harper Collins, 2007.

Bereiter, L. "Toward a Solution of the Learning Paradox." *Review of Educational Research* 55 (1985): 201–25.

Berninger, V., A. Chen, and R. Abbot. "A Test of the Multiple Connections Model of Reading Acquisition." *International Journal of Neuroscience* 42 (1988): 283–95.

Bishop, J. H. "Why the Apathy in American High Schools?" *Educational Researcher* 18, no. 1 (1989): 6–10.

Block, N., and G. Dworkin. *The I.Q. Controversy*. New York: Pantheon, 1976.

Bloom, B. S. "The Z Sigma Problem: The Search for Methods of Group Instruction as Effective as One-to-One Tutoring." *Educational Researcher* 13, no. 6 (1984): 4–16.

Bloom, F. E., M. F. Beal, and D. J. Kupfer, eds. *The Dana Guide to Brain Health: A Practical Family Guide from Medical Experts*. New York: Dana Press, 2003.

Boller, K., and C. Rovee-Collier. "Contextual Coding and Recording of Infants' Memories." *Journal of Experimental Child Psychology* 53, no. 1 (1992): 1–23.

Borkowski, J. G., W. Schneider, and M. Pressley. "The Challenges of Teaching Good Information Processing to the Learning Disabled Student." *International Journal of Disability, Development and Education* 3, no. 3 (1989): 169–85.

Botha, L. "SALT in Practice: A Report on Progress." *Journal of the Society for Accelerative Learning and Teaching* 10, no. 3 (1985): 197–99.

Botkin, J. W., M. Elmandjra, and M. Malitza. *No Limits to Learning: Bridging the Human Gap: A Report of the Club of Rome*. Oxford: Pergammon Press, 1979.

Boyle, P. "Having a Higher Purpose in Life Reduces Risk of Death among Older Adults." *Science Daily*, June 18, 2009. http://www.sciencedaily.com/releases/2009/06/090615144207.htm.

Brain and Mind Symposium. Columbia University. May 13–14, 2004. http://c250.co lumbia.edu/c250_events/symposia/brain_mind/brain_mind_vid_archive.html.

Bransford, J. D. *Human Cognition*. Belmont, CA: Wadsworth, 1979.

Braten, I. "Vygotsky as Precursor to Metacognitive Theory, II: Vygotsky as Metacognitivist." *Scandinavian Journal of Educational Research* 35, no. 4 (1991): 305–20.

Briggs, M. H. "Team Talk: Communication Skills for Early Intervention Teams." *Journal of Childhood Communication Disorders* 15, no. 1 (1993): 33–40.

Broadbent, D. E. *Perception and Communication*. London: Pergammon Press, 1958.

Brown, A. L. "Knowing When, Where and How to Remember: A Problem of Meta-Cognition." In *Advances in Instructional Psychology*. Edited by R. Glaser. Hillsdale, NJ: Melbourne, 1978.

Bunker, V. J., W. M. McBurnett, and D. L. Fenimore. "Integrating Language Intervention throughout the School Community." *Journal of Childhood Communication Disorders* 11, no. 1 (1987): 185–92.

Buzan, T. *Head First*. London: Thorsons, 2000.

———. *Use Both Sides of Your Brain*. New York: Plume, 1991.

Buzan, T., and R. Keene. *The Age Heresy*. London: Ebury Press, 1996.

Bynum, J. *Matters of the Heart*. Lake Mary, FL: Charisma House, 2002.

Byron, R. *Behaviour in Organisations: Understanding and Managing the Human Side of Work*. 2nd ed. Boston: Allyn and Bacon, 1986.

Byron, R., and D. Byrne. *Social Psychology: Understanding Human Interaction*. 4th ed. Boston: Allyn and Bacon, 1984.

Calvin, W., and G. Ojemann. *Conversations with Neil's Brain*. Reading, MA: Addison-Wesley, 1994.

Campbell, B., L. Campbell, and D. Dickinson. *Teaching and Learning through Multiple Intelligences*. Seattle: New Horizons for Learning, 1992.

Campione, J. C., A. L. Brown, and N. R. Bryant. "Individual Differences in Learning and Memory." In *Human Abilities: An Information Processing Approach*. Edited by R. J. Sternberg. New York: West Freeman, 1984, 103–26.

Cantor, C. "Rutgers-Newark Program Aims to Combat Alzheimer's Disease in Black Communities." *Rutgers Focus*. March 26, 2008. http://news.rutgers.edu/focus/issue.2008-03-26.6300207636/article.2008-03-26.8293146433.

Capra, F. "The Turning Point: A New Vision of Reality." *The Futurist* 16 no. 6 (1982): 19–24.

Caskey, O. "Accelerating Concept Formation." *Journal of the Society for Accelerative Learning and Teaching* 11, no. 3 (1986): 137–45.

Chi, M. "Interactive Roles of Knowledge and Strategies in the Development of Organized Sorting and Recall." In *Thinking and Learning Skills*, vol. 2. Edited by S. F. Chipman, J. W. Segal, and R. Glaser. Hillsdale, NJ: Lawrence Erlbaum, 1985.

Childre, D., and H. Martin. *The Heartmath Solution*. San Francisco: HarperCollins, 1999.

Church, D. *The Genie in Your Genes*. Fulton, CA: Energy Psychology Press, 2008.

Clancey, W. "Why Today's Computers Don't Learn the Way People Do." Paper presented at the Annual Meeting of the American Educational Research Association, Boston, 1990.

Clark, A. J. "Forgiveness: A Neurological Model." *Medical Hypotheses* 65 (2005): 649–54.

Colbert, D. *The Bible Cure for Memory Loss*. Lake Mary, FL: Siloam Press, 2001.

———. *Deadly Emotions: Understand the Mind-Body-Spirit Connection That Can Heal or Destroy You*. Nashville: Thomas Nelson, 2003.

Cook, N. D. "Collosal Inhibition: The Key to the Brain Code." *Behavioral Science* 29 (1984): 98–110.

Costa, A. L. "Mediating the Metacognitive." *Educational Leadership* 42, no. 3 (1984): 57–62.

Cousins, N. *Anatomy of an Illness as Perceived by the Patient.* New York: Bantam, 1981.

———. "Anatomy of an Illness as Perceived by the Patient." *New England Journal of Medicine* 295 (1976): 1458–63.

Crick, F. *The Astonishing Hypothesis: The Scientific Search for the Soul.* New York: Scribner, 1995.

———. "Thinking about the Brain." *Scientific American* 241, no. 3 (1981): 228.

Cromie, W. J. "Childhood Abuse Hurts the Brain." *Harvard University Gazette.* http://news.harvard.edu/gazette/2003/05.22/01-brain.html.

———. "Research Links Sleep, Dreams, and Learning." *Harvard University Gazette.* www.news.harvard.edu/gazette/1996/02.08/ResearchLinksSl.html.

Damasio, A. R. *The Feeling of What Happens: Body and Motion in the Making of Consciousness.* New York: Harcourt, Brace, 1999.

Damico, J. S. "Addressing Language Concerns in the Schools: The SLP as Consultant." *Journal of Childhood Communication Disorders* 11, no. 1 (1987): 17–40.

Dartigues, J. F. "Use It or Lose It." *Omni,* February 1994, 34.

De Andrade, L. M. "Intelligence's Secret: The Limbic System and How to Mobilize It through Suggestopedy." *Journal of the Society for Accelerative Learning and Teaching* 11, no. 2 (1986): 103–13.

De Capdevielle, B. "An Overview of Project Intelligence." *Per Linguam* 2, no. 2 (1986): 31–38.

Decety, J., and J. Grezes. "Neural Mechanisms Subserving the Perception of Human Actions." *Trends in Cognitive Sciences* 3, no. 5 (May 1999): 172–78. http://condor.depaul.edu/dallbrit/extra/psy588/Decety-Grezes.pdf.

———. "The Power of Simulation: Imagining One's Own and Other's Behavior." *Brain Research* 1079 (2006): 4–14.

Decety, J., and P. L. Jackson. "A Social Neuroscience Perspective of Empathy." *Current Directions in Psychological Science* 15 (2006): 54–58.

Derry, S. J. "Remediating Academic Difficulties through Strategy Training: The Acquisition of Useful Knowledge." *Remedial and Special Education* 11, no. 6 (1990): 19–31.

Dhority, L. *The ACT Approach: The Artful Use of Suggestion for Integrative Learning.* Bremen, West Germany: PLS Verlag, An derWeide, 1991.

Diamond, M. *Enriching Heredity: The Impact of the Environment on the Brain.* New York: Free Press, 1988.

Diamond, M., and J. Hopson. *Magic Trees of the Mind: How to Nurture Your Child's Intelligence, Creativity, and Healthy Emotions from Birth through Adolescence.* New York: Penguin, 1999.

Diamond, S., and J. Beaumont, eds. *Hemisphere Function of the Human Brain.* London: Elek, 1974, 264–78.

Dienstbier, R. "Periodic Adrenalin Arousal Boosts Health Coping." *Brain-Mind Bulletin* 14, no. 9a (1989).

Dispenza, J. *Breaking the Habit of Being Yourself*. New York: Hay House, 2012.

———. *Evolve Your Brain: The Science of Changing Your Brain*. Deerfield Beach, FL: Health Communications, 2007.

Dixon, T., and T. Buzan. *The Evolving Brain*. Exetar, UK: Wheaten, 1976.

Dobson, J. *The New Hide or Seek: Self-Confidence in Your Child*. Grand Rapids: Revell, 1999.

Doidge, N. *The Brain That Changes Itself: Stories of Personal Triumph from the Frontiers of Brain Science*. New York: Penguin Books, 2007.

Dukas, H., and B. Hoffman. *Albert Einstein, the Human Side: New Glimpses from His Archives*. Princeton, NJ: Princeton University Press, 1979.

"Dwelling On Stressful Events Can Create Inflammation in the Body, Study Finds." *Science Daily*. March 13, 2013. http://www.sciencedaily.com/releases /2013/03/130313182255.htm?utm_source=feedburner&utm_medium=email &utm_campaign=Feed%3A+sciencedaily+%28ScienceDaily%3A+Latest +Science+News%29.

Edelman, G. M., and V. B. Mountcastle, eds. *The Mindful Brain*. Cambridge, MA: MIT Press, 1982.

Edelman, G. M., and G. Tononi. *A Universe of Consciousness: How Matter Becomes Imagination*. New York: Basic Books, 2000.

Edwards, B. *Drawing on the Right Side of the Brain*. Los Angeles: J. P. Torcher, 1979.

Ende, R. N. *Rene A. Spitz: Dialogues from Infancy*. Madison, CT: International Universities Press, 1984.

Entwistle, N. "Motivational Factors in Students' Approaches in Learning." In *Learning Strategies and Learning Styles*. Edited by R. R. Schmeck. New York: Plenum, 1988, 21–51.

Entwistle, N. J., and P. Ramsdon. *Understanding Student Learning*. London: Croom Helm, 1983.

"Epigenetics: http://www.docstoc.com/docs/129237704/Introduction-to-Epigenetics.

Eriksen, C. W., and J. Botella. "Filtering versus Parallel Processing in RSVP Tasks." *Perception and Psychophysics* 51, no. 4 (1992): 334–43.

Erskine, R. "A Suggestopedic Math Project Using Non-Learning Disabled Students." *Journal of the Society for Accelerative Learning and Teaching* 11, no. 4 (1986): 225–47.

Farah, M. J., F. Peronnet, L. L. Weisberg, and M. Monheit. "Brain Activity Underlying Visual Imagery: Event Related Potentials During Mental Image Generation." *Journal of Cognitive Neuroscience* 1 (1990): 302–16.

Faure, C. *Learning to Be: The World of Education Today and Tomorrow*. Paris: UNESCO, 1972.

Feldman, D. *Beyond Universals in Cognitive Development*. Norwood, NJ: Ablex, 1980.

Feuerstein, R. *Instrumental Enrichment: An Intervention Programme for Cognitive Modifiability*. Baltimore: University Park Press, 1980.

Feuerstein, R., M. Jensen, S. Roniel, and N. Shachor. "Learning Potential Assessment." *Assessment of Exceptional Children*. Haworth Press, 1986.

"Five for 2005: Five Reasons to Forgive." *Harvard Health Publications Newsletter* 2, no. 5 (January 15, 2005). http://harvardhealth.staywell.com/viewNewsletter.aspx?NLID=30&INC=yes.

Flavell, J. H. "Metacognitive Development." In *Structural/Process Theories of Complete Human Behaviour*. Edited by J. M. Scandura and C. J. Brainerd. Alphen aan den Rijn, The Netherlands: Sijthoff and Noordoff, 1978.

Flavell, P. *The Developmental Psychology of Jean Piaget*. New York: Basic Books, 1963.

Fodor, J. *The Modularity of Mind*. Cambridge, MA: MIT/Bradford, 1983.

Fountain, D. *God, Medicine, and Miracles: The Spiritual Factors in Healing*. New York: Random House, 2000.

Frassinelli, L., K. Superior, and J. Meyers. "A Consultation Model for Speech and Language Intervention." *ASHA* 25 no. 4 (1983): 25–30.

Freeman, W. J. *Societies of Brains: A Study in the Neuroscience of Love and Hate*. Hillsdale, NJ: Lawrence Erlbaum Associates, 1995.

"Free Tools to Help You Cope with Stress." *Harvard Health Publications*. Harvard Medical School. www.health.harvard.edu/topic/stress.

Galton, F. *Inquiries into Human Faculty and Its Development*. London: L. M. Dent, 1907.

Gardner, H. *Frames of Mind*. New York: Basic Books, 1985.

———. *The Quest for Mind: Piaget, Levi-Strauss, and the Structuralist Movement*. Chicago: University of Chicago Press, 1981.

Gardner, H., and D.P. Wolfe. "Waves and Streams of Symbolization." In *The Acquisition of Symbolic Skills*. Edited by D. Rogers and J. A. Slabada. London: Plenum Press, 1983.

Gazzaniga, M. S. *Handbook of Neuropsychology*. New York: Plenum, 1977.

———, ed. *The New Cognitive Neurosciences*. Cambridge, MA: MIT/Bradford, 2004.

Gelb, M. *Present Yourself*. Los Angeles: Jalmar Press, 1988.

Gerber, A. "Collaboration between SLP's and Educators: A Continuity Education Process." *Journal of Childhood Communication Disorders* 11, no. 1–2 (1987): 107–25.

"Ghost in Your Genes." PBS NOVA. www.pbs.org/wgbh/nova/genes.

Glaser, R. *Adaptive Education: Individual Diversity and Learning*. New York: Holt, Rhinehart and Winston, 1977.

Glasser, M. D. *Control Theory in the Classroom*. New York: Harper & Row, 1986.

Goldberg, E., and L. D. Costa. "Hemisphere Differences in the Acquisition and Use of Descriptive Systems." *Brain and Language* 14 (1981):144–73.

Golden, F. "Albert Einstein: Person of the Century." *Time*, December 31, 1999.

Gould, S. "Commission on Nontraditional Study." *Diversity by Design*. San Francisco: Jossey-Bass, 1973.

———. *The Mismeasure of Man*. New York: Norton, 1981.

Griffiths, D. E. "Behavioural Science and Educational Administration." In *63rd Yearbook of the National Society for the Study of Education*. Chicago: NSSE, 1964.

Gungor, E. *There Is More to the Secret*. Nashville: Thomas Nelson, 2007.

Guse, J. "How the Marx Brothers Brought Norman Cousins Back to Life." *The Healing Power of Laughter*. http://thehealingpoweroflaughter.blogspot.com/2007/07/how-marx-brothers-brought-norman.html.

Guyton, A. C., and J. E. Halle. *Textbook of Medical Physiology*. 9th ed. Philadelphia: W. D. Saunders, 1996.

Haber, R. N. "The Power of Visual Perceiving." *Journal of Mental Imagery 5* (1981): 1–40.

Halpern, S., and L. Savary. *Sound Health: The Music and Sounds That Make Us Whole*. San Francisco: Harper & Row, 1985.

Hamilton, P. J., D. J. Furman, C. Chang, M. E. Thomason, E. Dennis, and I. H. Gotlib. "Default-Mode and Task-Positive Network Activity in Major Depressive Disorder: Implications for Adaptive and Maladaptive Rumination." *Biological Psychiatry* 70, no. 4 (2011): 327–33.

Hand, J. D. "The Brain and Accelerative Learning." *Per Linguam* 2, no. 2 (1986): 2–14.

Hand, J. D., and B. L. Stein. "The Brain and Accelerative Learning, Part II: The Brain and Its Functions." *Journal of the Society for Accelerative Learning and Teaching* 11, no. 3 (1986): 149–63.

Harlow, H. Databank Entry in "People and Discoveries: Harry Harlow." *PBS: A Science Odyssey*. www.pbs.org/wgbh/aso/databank/entries/bhharl.html.

Harrell, K. D. *Attitude Is Everything: A Tune-Up to Enhance Your Life*. Dubuque, IA: Kendall Hunt, 1995.

Harrison, C. J. "Metacognition and Motivation." *Reading Improvement* 28, no. 1 (1993): 35–39.

Hart, L. *Human Brain and Human Learning*. New York: Longman, 1983.

Hatfied, R. W. "Touch and Human Sexuality." In *Human Sexuality: An Encyclopedia*. Edited by V. Bullough, B. Bullough, and A. Stein. New York: Garland, 1994.

Hatton, G. I. "Function-Related Plasticity in the Hypothalamus." *Annual Review of Neuroscience* 20 (1997): 375–97.

Hawkins, D. B. *When Life Makes You Nervous: New and Effective Treatments for Anxiety*. Colorado Springs: Cook, 2001.

Hayman, J. L. "Systems Theory and Human Organization." In *A Systems Approach to Learning Environments*. Edited by S. D. Zalatimo and P. J. Steeman. Roselle, NJ: MEDED Projects, 1975.

"The Health Benefits of Laughter." http://heyugly.org/LaughterOneSheet2.php.

Healy, J. "Why Kids Can't Think: Bottom Line." *Personal* 13, no. 8 (1993): 1–3.

Hinton, G .E., and J. A. Anderson. *Parallel Models of Associative Memory*. Hillsdale, NJ: Erlbaum, 1981.

Hochberg, L. R., M. D. Serruya, G. M. Friehs, J. A. Mukand, M. Saleh, A. H. Caplan, A. Branner, D. Chen, R. D. Penn, and J .P. Donoghue. "Neuronal Ensemble Control of Prosthetic Devices by a Human with Tetraplegia." *Nature* 442, no. 7099 (July 18, 2006): 164–71.

Holden, C. "Child Development: Small Refugees Suffer the Effects of Early Neglect." *Science* 305 (1996):1076–77.

Holford, P. *How Children Fail*. New York: Pitman, 1964.

———. *The Optimum Nutrition Bible*. London: Piatkus, 1997.

———. *Optimum Nutrition for the Mind*. London: Piatkus, 2003.

———. *The 30-Day Fat Burner Diet*. London: Piatkus, 1999.

Hubel, D. H. "The Brain." *Scientific American* 24, no. 13 (1979): 45–53.

Hunter, C., F. Hunter, and F. Contreras. *Laugh Yourself Healthy—Keep the Doctor Away with a Giggle a Day*. Lake Mary, FL: Christian Life, 2008.

Hyden, H. "The Differentiation of Brain Cell Protein, Learning, and Memory." *Biosystems* 8, no. 4 (1977): 22–30.

Hyman, S. E. "Addiction: A Disease of Learning and Memory." *American Journal of Psychiatry* 162 (2005): 1414–22.

Iaccino, J. *Left Brain–Right Brain Differences: Inquiries, Evidence, and New Approaches*. Hillsdale, NJ: Erlbaum, 1993.

Institute of HeartMath. www.heartmath.org/research/science-of-the-heart.html.

Iran-Nejad, A. "Active and Dynamic Self-Regulation of Learning Processes." *Review of Educational Research* 60, no. 4 (1990): 573–602.

———. "Associative and Nonassociative Schema Theories of Learning." *Bulletin of the Psychonomic Society* 27 (1989): 1–4.

———. "The Schema: A Long-Term Memory Structure or a Transient Functional Pattern." In *Understanding Reader's Understanding*. Edited by R. J. Teireny, P. L. Anders, and J. N. Mitchell. Hillsdale, NJ: Erlbaum, 1987, 109–28.

Iran-Nejad, A., and B. Chissom. "Active and Dynamic Sources of Self-Regulation." Paper presented at the Annual Meeting of the American Psychological Association, Atlanta, Georgia, 1988.

Iran-Nejad, A., and A. Ortony. "A Biofunctional Model of Distributed Mental Content, Mental Structures, Awareness and Attention." *Journal of Mind and Behavior* 5 (1984): 171–210.

Iran-Nejad, A., A. Ortony, and R. K. Rittenhouse. "The Comprehension of Metaphonical Uses of English by Deaf Children." *American Speech-Language-Association* 24 (1989): 551–56.

Jacobs, B., M. Schall, and A. B. Scheibel. "A Quantitative Dendritic Analysis of Wernickes Area in Humans: Gender, Hemispheric and Environmental Factors." *Journal of Comparative Neurology* 327, no. 1 (1993): 97–111.

Jensen, A. *Bias in Mental Testing*. New York: Free Press, 1980.

Jensen, E. *Brain-Based Learning and Teaching*. Johannesburg, South Africa: Process Graphix, 1995.

Johnson, D. W., R. T. Johnson, and E. Holubec. *Circles of Learning: Cooperation in the Classroom*. Edina, MN: Interaction Books, 1986.

Johnson, J. M. "A Case History of Professional Evolution from SLP to Communication Instructor." *Journal of Childhood Communication Disorders* 11, no. 4 (1987): 225–34.

Jorgensen, C. C., and W. Kintsch. "The Role of Imagery in the Evaluation of Sentences." *Cognitive Psychology* 4 (1973): 110–16.

Kagan, A, and M. M. Saling. *An Introduction to Luria's Aphasiology Theory and Application*. Johannesburg, South Africa: Witwatersrand University Press, 1988.

Kalivas, P. W., and N. Volkow. "The Neural Basis of Addiction: A Pathology of Motivation and Choice." *American Journal of Psychiatry* 162 (2005): 1403–13.

Kandel, E. R. *In Search of Memory: The Emergence of a New Science of Mind*. New York: W. W. Norton, 2006.

———. "The Molecular Biology of Memory Storage: A Dialog between Genes and Synapses." Nobel Lecture. December 8, 2000. www.nobelprize.org/nobel_prizes/medicine/laureates/2000/kandel-lecture.pdf.

———. "A New Intellectual Framework for Psychiatry." *American Journal of Psychiatry* 155, no. 4 (1998): 457–69.

Kandel, E. R, J. H. Schwartz, and T. M. Jessell, eds. *Essentials of Neural Science and Behavior*. New York: Appleton and Lange, 1995.

———, eds. *Principles of Neural Science*. 4th ed. New York: McGraw-Hill, 2000.

Kaniels, S., and R. Feuerstein. "Special Needs of Children with Learning Difficulties." *Oxford Review of Education* 15, no. 2 (1989): 165–79.

Kaplan-Solms, K., and M. Sloms. *Clinical Studies in Neuro-Psychoanalysis*. New York: Karnac, 2002.

Kazdin, A. E. "Covert Modelling, Imagery Assessment and Assertive Behaviour." *Journal of Consulting and Clinical Psychology* 43 (1975): 716–24.

Kimara, D. "The Assymmetry of the Human Brain." *Scientific American* 228, no. 3 (1973): 70–80.

———. "Sex Differences in the Brain." *Scientific American* 267, no. 3 (September 1992): 119–25.

King, D. F., and K. S. Goodman. "Whole Language Learning, Cherishing Learners and their Language." *Language, Speech and Hearing Sciences in Schools*, 21 (1990): 221–29.

Kintsch, W. "Learning from Text, Levels of Comprehension, or: Why Anyone Would Read a Story Anyway?" *Poetics* 9, 1980, 87–98.

Kline, P. *Everyday Genius*. Arlington, VA: Great Ocean Publishers, 1990.

Kluger, J. "The Biology of Belief." *Time*, February 12, 2009. www.time.com/time/health/article/0,8599,1879016,00.html.

Knowles, M. *The Adult Learner: A Neglected Species*. Houston: Gulf Publishing, 1990.

Konnikova, M. *Mastermind*. New York: Viking, 2013.

———. "The Power of Concentration." *New York Times Sunday Review*. December 15, 2012. www.nytimes.com/2012/12/16/opinion/sunday/the-power-of-concentration.html?pagewanted=1&_r=2&ref=general&src=me&.

Kopp, M. S., and J. Rethelyi. "Where Psychology Meets Physiology: Chronic Stress and Premature Mortality: The Central–Eastern European Health Paradox." *Brain Research Bulletin* 62 (2004): 351–67.

Kosslyn, S. M., and O. Koenig. *Wet Mind: The New Cognitive Neuroscience*. New York: Free Press, 1995.

Kubzansky, L. D., I. Kawachi, A. Spiro III, S. T. Weiss, P. S. Vokonas, and D. Sparrow. "Is Worrying Bad for Your Heart? A Prospective Study of Worry and Coronary Heart Disease in the Normative Aging Study." *Circulation* 94, no. 4. (1997): 818–24.

Lahaye, T., and D. Noebel. *Mind Siege: The Battle for Truth in the New Millennium*. Nashville: Word, 2000.

Lally, P., C. H. M. van Jaarsveld, H. W. W. Potts, and J. Wardle. "How Are Habits Formed: Modelling Habit Formation in the Real World." *European Journal of Social Psychology* 40, no. 6 (2009): 998–1009.

Langer, E., and M. Moldoveanu. "The Construct of Mindfulness." *Journal of Social Issue* 56, no. 1 (2000): 1–9.

Larsson, G., and B. Starrin. "Effect of Relaxation Training on Verbal Ability, Sequential Thinking and Spatial Ability." *Journal of the Society of Accelerative Learning and Teaching* 13, no. 2 (1988): 147–59.

Lazar, C. "A Review and Appraisal of Current Information on Speech/Language Alternative Service Delivery Models in Schools." *Communiphon* 308 (1994): 8–11.

Lazar, S. W., and C. E. Kerr. "Meditation Experience Is Associated with Increased Cortical Thickness." *NeuroReport* 16, no. 17 (2005): 189–97.

Lea, L. *Wisdom: Don't Live Life without It*. Guilford, Surrey, UK: Highland Books, 1980.

Leaf, C. M. "An Altered Perception of Learning: Geodesic Learning." *Therapy Africa* 1, no. 2 (October 1997): 7.

———. "An Altered Perception of Learning: Geodesic Learning: Part 2." *Therapy Africa* 2, no. 1 (January/February 1998): 4.

———. "The Development of a Model for Geodesic Learning: The Geodesic Information Processing Model." *The South African Journal of Communication Disorders* 44, (1997): 53–70.

———. "Evaluation and Remediation of High School Children's Problems Using the Mind Mapping Therapeutic Approach." *Remedial Teaching* 7/8, University of South Africa (September 1992).

———. "The Mind Mapping Approach: A Model and Framework for Geodesic Learning." Unpublished DPhil. dissertation, University of Pretoria, South Africa, 1997.

———. "The Mind Mapping Approach (MMA): Open the Door to Your Brain Power: Learn How to Learn." *Transvaal Association of Educators Journal* (December 1992).

———. "The Mind Mapping Approach: A Technique for Closed Head Injury." Unpublished master's dissertation, University of Pretoria, South Africa.

———. "Mind Mapping as a Therapeutic Intervention Technique." Unpublished workshop manual, 1985.

———. "Mind Mapping as a Therapeutic Technique." *Communiphon* 296 (1989): 11–15. A publication of the South African Speech-Language-Hearing Association.

———. "The Move from Institution Based Rehabilitation (IBR) to Community Based Rehabilitation (CBR): A Paradigm Shift." *Therapy Africa* 1, no. 1 (August 1997): 4.

———. *Switch On Your Brain 5-Step Learning Process.* Dallas: Switch on Your Brain, 2008.

———. *Switch On Your Brain: Understand Your Unique Intelligence Profile and Maximize Your Potential.* Cape Town, South Africa: Tafelberg, 2005.

———. *Switch On Your Brain with the Metacognitive-Mapping Approach.* Elkhart, IN: Truth Publishing, 2002.

———. "Teaching Children to Make the Most of Their Minds: Mind Mapping." *Journal for Technical and Vocational Education in South Africa* 121 (1990): 11–13.

———. *Who Switched Off My Brain? Controlling Toxic Thoughts and Emotions.* Dallas: Switch on Your Brain, 2007.

———. "Who Switched Off My Brain? Controlling Toxic Thoughts and Emotions." DVD series. Johannesburg, South Africa: Switch On Your Brain, 2007.

Leaf, C. M., M. Copeland, and J. Maccaro. "Your Body His Temple: God's Plan for Achieving Emotional Wholeness." DVD series. Dallas: Life Outreach International, 2007.

Leaf, C. M., I. C. Uys, and B. Louw. "An Alternative Non-Traditional Approach to Learning: The Metacognitive-Mapping Approach." *The South African Journal of Communication Disorders* 45 (1998): 87–102.

———. "The Development of a Model for Geodesic Learning: The Geodesic Information Processing Model." *The South African Journal for Communication Disorders* 44 (1997).

———. "The Mind Mapping Approach (MMA): A Culture and Language-Free Technique." *The South African Journal of Communication Disorders* 40 (1992): 35–43.

LeDoux, J. *Synaptic Self: How Our Brains Become Who We Are.* New York: Penguin, 2002.

Leedy, P. D. *Practical Research: Planning and Design.* New York: Macmillan, 1989.

Lehmann, E. L. *Non-Parametric: Statistical Methods Based on Ranks.* San Francisco: Holden-Day, 1975.

Leuchter, A. F., I. A. Cook, E. A. Witte, M. Morgan, and M. Abrams. "Changes in Brain Function of Depressed Subjects During Treatment with Placebo." *American Journal of Psychiatry* 159, no. 1 (2002): 122–29.

Levy, J. "Interview." *Omni* 7, no. 4 (1985).

———. "Research Synthesis on Right and Left Hemispheres: We Think with Both Sides of the Brain." *Educational Leadership* 40, no. 4 (1983): 66–71.

Lewis, R. "Report Back on the Workshop: Speech/Language/Hearing Therapy in Transition." *Communiphon* 308 (1994): 6–7.

Liebertz, C. "Want Clear Thinking: Relax." *Scientific American* (September 21, 2005). www.scientificamerican.com/article.cfm?id=want-clear-thinking-relax.

Lipton, B. *The Biology of Belief: Unleashing the Power of Consciousness, Matter and Miracles.* Santa Cruz, CA: Mountain of Love Productions, 2008.

Lipton, B. H., K. G. Bensch, and M. A. Karasek. "Microvessel Endothelial Cell Transdifferentiation: Phenotypic Characterization." *Differentiation* 46, no. 2 (1991): 117–33.

Llinas, R. *I of the Vortex.* Cambridge, MA: MIT Press, 2002.

Lozanov, G. *Suggestology and Outlines of Suggestopedy.* New York: Gordon and Breach Science Publishers, 1978.

Lozanov, G., and G. Gateva. *The Foreign Language Educator's Suggestopaedic Manual.* New York: Gordon and Breach Science Publishers, 1989.

L. T. F. A. "Brain-Based Learning." Unpublished lecture series. Johannesburg, South Africa: Lead the Field Africa, 1995.

Luria, A .R. *Higher Cortical Functions in Man.* 2nd ed. New York: Basic Books, 1980.

Lutz, K. A., and J. W. Rigney. *The Memory Book.* New York: Skin and Day, 1977.

MacLean, P. "A Mind of Three Minds: Educating the Triune Brain." *77th Yearbook of the National Society for the Study of Education.* Chicago: University of Chicago Press, 1978, 308–42.

Margulies, N. *Mapping Inner-Space.* Tucson, AZ: Zephyr Press, 1991.

Markram, H. "'Blue Brain' Project Accurately Predicts Connections between Neurons." *ScienceDaily* (September 17, 2012). Reprinted from materials provided by Ecole Polytechnique Fédérale de Lausanne. www.sciencedaily.com/releases/2012/09/120917152043.htm.

Marvin, C. A. "Consultation Services: Changing Roles for the SLP's." *Journal of Childhood Communication Disorders* 11, no. 1 (1987): 1–15.

Maslow, A. H. *Motivation and Personality.* New York: Harper & Row, 1970.

Mastropieri, M. A., and J. P. Bakken. "Applications of Metacognition." *Remedial and Special Education* 11, no. 6 (1990): 32–35.

Matheny, K. B., and J. McCarthy. *Prescription for Stress.* Oakland, CA: New Harbinger Publications, 2000.

McAllister, A. K. "Cellular and Molecular Mechanisms of Dendritic Growth." *Cerebral Cortex* 10, no. 10 (2000): 963–73.

McEwan, B. S. "Stress and Hippocampal Plasticity." *Annual Review of Neuroscience* 22 (1999): 105–22.

McEwan, B. S., and E. N. Lasley. *The End of Stress as We Know It.* Washington, DC: National Academies Press, 2002.

McEwan, B. S., and T. Seeman. "Protective and Damaging Effects of Mediators of Stress: Elaborating and Testing the Concepts of Allostasis and Allostatic Load." *Annals of the New York Academy of Science* 896 (1999): 30–47.

McGaugh, J. L., and I. B. Intrioni-Collision. "Involvement of the Amygdaloidal Complex in Neuromodulatory Influences on Memory Storage." *Neuroscience and Behavioural Reviews* 14, no. 4 (1990): 425–31.

"Meditation's Positive Residual Effects: Imaging Finds Different Forms of Meditation May Affect Brain Structure." *Harvard Gazette.* http://news.harvard.edu/gazette/story/2012/11/meditations-positive-residual-effects.

Merzenich, M. M. "Cortical Plasticity Contributing to Childhood Development." In *Mechanisms of Cognitive Development: Behavioral and Neural Perspectives.* Edited by J. L. McClelland and R. S. Siegler. Mahwah, NJ: Lawrence Erlbaum, 2001.

———. "Promising Results in Controlling Tinnitus with Brain Training." http://merzenich.positscience.com.

Meyer, J. *The Battlefield of the Mind: Winning the Battle in Your Mind.* New York: Faith Words, 1995.

———. *Life without Strife: How God Can Heal and Restore Troubled Relationships.* Lake Mary, FL: Charisma House, 2000.

Miller, G. A. "The Magical Number Seven, Plus or Minus Two: Some Limits on Our Capacity for Processing Information." *Psychological Review* 63 (1956): 81–97.

Miller, T., and D. Sabatino. "An Evaluation of the Educator Consultant Model as an Approach to Main Streaming." *Exceptional Children* 45 (1978).

"Mind/Body Connection: How Emotions Affect Your Health." FamilyDoctor.org. http://familydoctor.org/online/famdocen/home/healthy/mental/782.html.

Mogilner, A., J. A. Grossman, U. Ribary, M. Joliot, J. Volkmann, D. Rapaport, R. W. Beasley, and R. R. Llinas. "Somatosensory Cortical Plasticity in Adult Humans Revealed by Magnetoencephalography." *Proceedings of the National Academy of Sciences* 90, no. 8 (1993): 3593–97.

Montessori, M. *The Absorbent Mind.* Amsterdam: Clio Press, 1989.

Mountcastle, V. "An Organizing Principle for Cerebral Function: The Unit Module and the Distributed System." In *The Mindful Brain.* Edited by G. M. Edelman and V. Mountcastle. Cambridge, MA: MIT Press, 1978.

Nader, K. "Manipulating Memory." *MIT Technology Review.* www.technologyreview.com/video/413181/manipulating-memory.

Nader, K., G. E. Schafe, and J. E. Le Doux. "Fear Memories Require Protein Synthesis in the Amygdala for Reconsolidation after Retrieval." *Nature* 406, no. 6797 (2000): 722–26.

National Institute of Mental Health statistics. www.nimh.nih.gov/statistics/index. shtml.

Nelson, A. "Imagery's Physiological Base: The Limbic System: A Review Paper." *Journal of the Society for Accelerative Learning and Teaching* 13, no. 4 (1988): 363–71.

Nelson, R., ed. *Metacognition Core Readings*. Boston: Allyn and Bacon, 1992.

Newberg, A., E. D'Aquili, and V. Rause. *Why God Won't Go Away: Brain Science and the Biology of Belief*. New York: Ballantine, 2001.

Novak, J. D., B. Gowin, and J. B. Kahle. *Learning How to Learn*. Cambridge, UK: Cambridge University Press, 1984.

Nummela, R. M., and T. M. Rosengren. "Orchestration of Internal Processing." *Journal for the Society of Accelerated Learning and Teaching* 10, no. 2 (1985): 89–97.

Odendaal, M. S. "Needs Analysis of Higher Primary Educators in KwaZulu." *Per Linguam*, special issue no. 1 (1985): 5–99.

Okebukola, P. A. "Attitudes of Educators Towards Concept Mapping and Vee-Diagramming as Metalearning Tools in Science and Mathematics." *Educational Research* 34, no. 3 (1992): 201–12.

O'Keefe, J., and L. Nadel. *The Hippocampus as a Cognitive Map*. New York: Oxford University Press, 1978.

Olivier, C. *Let's Educate, Train and Learn Outcomes-Based: A 3D Experience in Creativity*. Pretoria, South Africa: Benedic, 1999.

Olsen, K. E. *Outcomes Based Education: An Experiment in Social Engineering*. Kranskop, South Africa: Christians for Truth. 1997.

O'Mathuna, D., and W. Larimore. *Alternative Medicine: The Christian Handbook*. Updated and expanded. Grand Rapids: Zondervan, 2007.

Ornstein, R. E. *The Psychology of Consciousness*. New York: Penguin Books, 1975.

Ornstein, R. *The Right Mind: Making Sense of the Hemispheres*. Orlando, FL: Harcourt, Brace, 1997.

Palincsar, A. S., and A. L. Brown. "Reciprocal Teaching of Comprehension Fostering and Monitoring Activities." *Cognition and Instruction* 1 (1984): 117–75.

Palmer, L. L., M. Alexander, and N. Ellis. "Elementary School Achievement Results Following In-Service Training of an Entire School Staff in Accelerative Learning and Teaching: An Interim Report." *Journal of the Society for Accelerative Learning and Teaching* 14, no. 1 (1989): 55–79.

Paris, S. G., and P. Winograd. "Promoting Metacognition and Motivation of Exceptional Children." *Remedial and Special Education* 11, no. 6 (1990): 7–15.

Pascuale-Leone, A., and R. Hamilton. "The Metamodal Organization of the Brain." In *Progress in Brain Research*. Edited by C. Casanova and M. Ptito (2001), 134.

Paul-Brown, D. "Professional Practices Perspective on Alternative Service Delivery Models." *ASHA Bulletin* 12 (1992).

Perlemutter, D., and C. Coleman. *The Better Brain Book*. New York: Penguin, 2004.

Pert, C. B. *Molecules of Emotion: Why You Feel the Way You Feel*. London: Simon and Schuster, 2004; New York: Simon and Schuster, 1999.

Pert, C., G. Pasternak, and S. H. Snyder. "Opiate Agonists and Antagonists Discriminated by Receptor Binding in the Brain." *Science* 182 (1973): 1359–61.

Peters, T. *Playing God? Genetic Determinism and Human Freedom*. 2nd ed. New York: Routledge, 2003.

Planck, M. "Max Planck Quotes." www.goodreads.com/author/quotes/107032. Max_Planck.

"The Pleasure Centres Affected by Drugs." *Canadian Institutes of Health Research*. http://thebrain.mcgill.ca/flash/i/i_03/i_03_cr/i_03_cr_par/i_03_cr_par.html.

Plotsky, P. M., and M.J. Meaney. "Early Postnatal Experience Alters Hypothalamic Corticotropin-Releasing Factor (CRF) mRNA, Median Eminence CRF Content and Stress-Induced Release in Adult Rats." *Molecular Brain Research* 18, no. 3 (1993): 195–200.

"Positive Psychology: Harnessing the Power of Happiness, Mindfulness, and Personal Strength." *Harvard Health Publications*. Harvard Medical School. www.health. harvard.edu/special_health_reports/positive-psychology-harnessing-the-power -of-happiness-personal-strength-and-mindfulness.

"Power of Forgiveness—Forgive Others." *Harvard Health Publications*. Harvard Medical School. December 2004. www.health.harvard.edu/press_releases/ power_of_forgiveness.

"The Prevalence of Mental Illness Today." *Harvard Health Publications*. Harvard Medical School. www.health.harvard.edu/newsweek/Prevalence-and-treatment-of-mental-illness-today.htm.

Pribram, K. H. *Languages of the Brain*. Monterey, CA: Brooks/Cole, 1971.

Pulvermuller, F. *The Neuroscience of Language: On Brain Circuits of Words and Serial Order*. Cambridge, UK: Cambridge University Press, 2002.

Raichle, M. E., A. M. MacLeod, A. Z. Snyder, W. J. Powers, D. A. Gusnard, and G. L. Shulman. "A Default Mode of Brain Function: A Brief History of an Evolving Idea." *Neuroimage* 37 (2007): 1083–90.

Rajechi, D. W. *Attitudes: Themes and Advances*. Sunderland, MA: Sinauer, 1982.

Ramachandran, V. S., and S. Blakeslee. *Phantoms in the Brain*. New York: William Morrow, 1998.

Redding, R. E. "Metacognitive Instruction: Trainers Teaching Thinking Skills." *Performance Improvement Quarterly* 3, no. 1 (1990): 27–41.

Restak, K. *The Brain: The Last Frontier*. New York: Doubleday, 1979.

Restak, R. *Mysteries of the Mind*. Washington, DC: National Geographic, 2000.

———. *Think Smart: A Neuroscientist's Prescription for Improving Your Brain Performance*. New York: Riverhead Books, 2009.

"Revised National Curriculum Statement Grades R-9." Policy document. Pretoria, South Africa: Department of Education, 2002.

Rizzolotti, G., and M. F. Destro. "Mirror Neurons." *Scholarpedia* 3, no. 1 (2008): 2055. http://www.scholarpedia.org/article/Mirror_neurons.

Rogers, C. R. *Freedom to Learn.* Columbus, OH: Merrill, 1969.

Rosenfield, I. *The Invention of Memory.* New York: Basic Books, 1988.

Rosenzweig, E. S., C. A. Barnes, and B. L. McNaughton. "Making Room for New Memories." *Nature Neuroscience* 5, no. 1 (2002): 6–8.

Rosenzweig, M. R., and E. L. Bennet. *Neuronal Mechanisms of Learning and Memory.* Cambridge, MA: MIT Press, 1976.

Rozin, P. "The Evolution of Intelligence and Access to the Cognitive Unconscious." *Progress in Psychobiology and Physiological Psychology* 6 (1975): 245–80.

Russell, P. *The Brain Book.* London: Routledge and Kegan Paul, 1986.

Rutherford, R., and K. Neethling. *Am I Clever or Am I Stupid?* Van-derbijlpark, South Africa: Carpe Diem Books, 2001.

Sagan, C. *The Dragons of Eden.* New York: Random House, 1977.

Saloman, G. *Interaction of Media, Cognition and Learning.* San Francisco: Jossey-Bass, 1979.

Samples, R. E. "Learning with the Whole Brain." *Human Behaviour* 4 (1975): 16–23.

Sapolsky, R. M. "Why Stress Is Bad for Your Brain." *Science* 273, no. 5276 (1996): 749–50.

Sarno, J. *The Mind-Body Prescription: Healing the Body, Healing the Pain.* New York: Werner Books, 1999.

Schallert, D. L. "The Significance of Knowledge: A Synthesis of Research Related to Schema Theory." In *Reading Expository Material.* Edited by W. Otto and S. White. New York: Academic, 1982, 13–48.

Schneider, W., and R. M. Shiffrin. "Controlled and Automatic Information Processing: I. Detection, Search and Attention." *Psychological Review* 88, no. 1 (1977): 1–66.

Schon, D. A. *Beyond the Stable State.* San Francisco: Jossey-Bass, 1971.

Schory, M. E. "Whole Language and the Speech Language Pathologists." *Language, Speech, and Hearing Services in Schools* 21 (1990): 206–11.

Schuster, D. H. "A Critical Review of American Foreign Language Studies Using Suggestopaedia." Paper delivered at the Aimav Linguistic Conference at the University of Nijmegen, the Netherlands, 1985.

Schwartz, J. M., and S. Begley. *The Mind and the Brain: Neuroplasticity and the Power of Mental Force.* New York: Regan Books/Harper Collins, 2002.

Schwartz, J. M., and R. Gladding. *You Are Not Your Brain.* New York: Avery, 2012.

Schwartz, J., H. Stapp, M. Beauregard. "Quantum Physics in Neuroscience and Psychology: A Neurophysical Model of Mind-Brain Interaction." *Philosophical Transactions of the Royal Society.* www.physics.lbl.gov/~stapp/PTB6.pdf.

Scruggs, E., and J. Brigham. "The Challenges of Metacognitive Instruction." *RASE* 11, no. 6 (1987): 16–18.

Seaward B. L. "Stress in America Today: Are Your Wellness Programs Prepared for the Super Stress Superstorm?" *Wellness Council of America News and Views,* 1996. www.brianlukeseaward.net/articles/SuperStress-WELCOA-Seaward.pdf.

Segerstrom, S. C., and G. E. Miller. "Psychological Stress and the Human Immune System: A Meta-Analytic Study of 30 Years of Inquiry." *Psychological Bulletin* 130, no. 4 (2004): 601–30.

Shapiro, R. B., V. G. Champagne, and D. De Costa "The Speech-Language Pathologist: Consultant to the Classroom Educator." *Reading Improvement* 25, no. 1 (1988): 2–9.

Shepard, B. "The Plastic Brain: Part 2." *UAB Magazine*. University of Alabama, Birmingham. www.uab.edu/uabmagazine/2009/may/plasticbrain2.

Sheth, B. R., D. Janvelyan, and M. Kahn. "Practice Makes Imperfect: Restorative Effects of Sleep on Motor Learning." *PLoS One* 3, no. 9 (2008): 3190.

Simon, C. S. "Out of the Broom Closet and into the Classroom: The Emerging SLP." *Journal of Childhood Communication Disorders* 11, no. 1–2 (1987): 81–90.

Singer, T., cited in Daniel Kane. "How Your Brain Handles Love and Pain." *NBC News: Science Mysteries*. www.msnbc.msn.com/id/4313263.

Sizer, T. R. *Horacel's Compromise: The Dilemma of the American High School*. Boston: Houghton Mifflin, 1984.

Slabbert, J. "Metalearning as the Most Essential Aim in Education for All." Paper presented at University of Pretoria, Faculty of Education, 1989.

Slife, B. D., J. Weiss, and T. Bell. "Separability of Metacognition and Cognition: Problem Solving in Learning Disabled and Regular Students." *Journal of Educational Psychology* 77, no. 4 (1985): 437–45.

Smith, A. *Accelerated Learning in Practice*. Stafford, UK: Network Educational Press, 1999.

Solms, M. "Forebrain Mechanisms of Dreaming Are Activated from a Variety of Sources." *Behavioral and Brain Sciences* 23, no. 6 (2000): 1035–40; 1083–1121.

Sperry, R. "Hemisphere Disconnection and Unity in Conscious Awareness." *American Psychologist* 23 (1968).

Springer, S. P., and G. Deutsch. *Left Brain, Right Brain*. New York: Freeman, 1998.

Sprouse, E. "5 Notable Discoveries in Epigenetics Research." http://dsc.discovery.com/tv-shows/curiosity/topics/5-discoveries-epigenetics-research.htm.

Stephan, K. M., G. R. Fink, R. E. Passingham, D. Silbersweig, A. O. Ceballos-Baumann, C. D. Firth, and R. S. J. Frackowiak. "Functional Anatomy of Mental Representation of Upper Extremity Movements in Healthy Subjects." *Journal of Neurophysiology* 73, no. 1 (1995): 373–86.

Sternberg, R. "The Nature of Mental Abilities." *American Psychologist* 34 (1979): 214–30.

Stickgold, R., J. A. Hobson, R. Fosse, and M. Fosse. "Sleep, Learning, and Dreams: Off-Line Memory Reprocessing." *Science* 294, no. 5554 (2001): 1052–57.

Stickgold, R., and P. Wehrwein. "Sleep Now, Remember Later." *Newsweek*, April 17, 2009. www.newsweek.com/id/194650.

Sylwester, R. "Research on Memory: Major Discoveries, Major Educational Challenges." *Educational Leadership* 42, no. 7 (1985): 69–75.

Tattershall, S. "Mission Impossible: Learning How a Classroom Works Before It's Too Late!" *Journal of Childhood Communication Disorders* 11, no. 1 (1987): 181–84.

Taub, E., G. Uswatte, M. Bowman, A. Delgado, C. Bryson, D. Morris, and V. W. Mark. "Use of CI Therapy for Plegic Hands after Chronic Stroke." Presentation at the Society for Neuroscience, Washington DC, November 16, 2005.

Taubes, G. *Good Calories, Bad Calories: Fats, Carbs and the Controversial Science of Diet and Health.* New York: Anchor Books, 2008.

Thembela, A. "Education for Blacks in South Africa: Issues, Problems and Perspectives." *Journal of the Society for Accelerative Learning and Teaching* 15, no. 1–2 (1990): 45–57.

Thurman, S. K., and A. H. Widerstrom. *Infants and Young Children with Special Needs: A Developmental and Ecological Approach.* 2nd ed. Baltimore: Paul H. Brookes, 1990.

Tunajek, S. "The Attitude Factor." Wellness Milestones. *AANA NewsBulletin,* April 2006. www.aana.com/resources2/health-wellness/Documents/nb_mile stone_0406.pdf.

Uys, I. C. "Single Case Experimental Designs: An Essential Service in Communicatively Disabled Care." *South African Journal of Communication Disorders* 36 (1989): 53–59.

Van derVyver, D. W. "SALT in South Africa: Needs and Parameters." *Journal of the Society for Accelerative Learning and Teaching* 10, no. 3 (1985): 187–200.

Van derVyver, D. W., and B. de Capdeville. "Towards the Mountain: Characteristics and Implications of the South African UPPTRAIL Pilot Project." *Journal of the Society for Accelerative Learning and Teaching* 15, no. 1–2 (1990): 59–74.

Van Praag, H., A. F. Schinder, B. R. Christie, N. Toni, T. D. Palmer, and F. H. Gage. "Functional Neurogenesis in the Adult Hippocampus." *Nature* 415, no. 6875 (2002): 1030–34.

Van Praag, H., B. L. Jacobs, and F. Gage. "Depression and the Birth and Death of Brain Cells." *American Scientist* 88, no. 4 (2000): 340–46.

Vaughan, S. C. *The Talking Cure: The Science Behind Psychotherapy.* New York: Grosset/Putnam, 1997.

Vaynman S., and E. Gomez-Pinilla. "License to Run: Exercise Impacts Functional Plasticity in the Intact and Injured Central Nervous System by Using Neurotrophins." *Neurorehabilitation and Neural Repair* 19, no. 4 (2005): 283–95.

Von Bertalanaffy, L. *General Systems Theory.* New York: Braziller, 1968.

Vythilingam, M., and C. Heim. "Childhood Trauma Associated with Smaller Hippocampal Volume in Women with Major Depression." *American Journal of Psychiatry* 159, no. 12 (2002): 2072–80.

Walker, M. P., and R. Stickgold. "Sleep, Memory and Plasticity." *Annual Review of Psychology* 57 (2006): 139–66.

Wark, D. M. "Using Imagery to Teach Study Skills." *Journal of the Society for Accelerative Learning and Teaching* 11, no. 3 (1986): 203–20.

Waterland, R. A., and R. L. Jirtle. "Transposable Elements: Targets for Early Nutritional Effects on Epigenetic Gene Regulation." *Molecular and Cellular Biology* 23, no. 15 (2003): 5293–300.

Watters, Ethan. "DNA Is Not Destiny: The New Science of Epigenetics Rewrites the Rules of Disease, Heredity, and Identity." *Discover: The Magazine of Science, Technology, and the Future*, November 2006. http://discovermagazine.com/2006/nov/cover.

Wenger, W. "An Example of Limbic Learning." *Journal of the Society for Accelerative Learning and Teaching* 10, no. 1 (1985): 51–68.

Wertsch, J. V. *Culture, Communication and Cognitions.* Cambridge, MA: Cambridge University Press, 1985.

Whitelson, S. "The Brain Connection: The Corpus Callosum Is Larger in Left-Handers." *Science* 229, no. 4714 (1985): 665–68.

Widener, C. *The Angel Inside: Michelangelo's Secrets for Following Your Passion and Finding the Work You Love.* New York: Crown Publishing, 2004.

Wiley, J., and A. F. Jarosz. "Working Memory Capacity, Attentional Focus, and Problem Solving." *Current Directions in Psychological Science* 21, no. 4 (2012): 258.

Wilson, R. S., C. F. Mendes De Leon, L. L. Barnes, J. A. Schneider, J. L. Bienias, D. A. Evans, and D. A. Bennett. "Participation in Cognitively Stimulating Activities and Risk of Incident Alzheimer Disease." *JAMA* 287, no. 6 (2002): 742–48.

Wright, N. H. *Finding Freedom from Your Fears.* Grand Rapids: Revell, 2005.

Wurtman, J. *Managing Your Mind and Mood through Food.* New York: Harper-Collins, 1986.

Young, L. J. "Being Human: Love: Neuroscience Reveals All." *Nature* 457, no. 148 (February 2009). www.nature.com/nature/journal/v457/n7226/full/457148a.html.

Zaidel, E. "Roger Sperry: An Appreciation." In *The Dual Brain.* Edited by D. F. Benson and E. Zaidel. New York: Guilford, 1985.

Zakaluk, B. L., and M. Klassen. "Enhancing the Performance of a High School Student Labelled Learning Disabled." *Journal of Reading* 36, no. 1 (1992).

Zdenek, M. *The Right Brain Experience.* Maidenhead, Berkshire, UK: McGraw-Hill, 1983.

Zimmerman, B. J., and D. H. Schunk. *Self-Regulated Learning and Academic Achievement: Theory, Research and Practice.* New York: Springer-Verby, 1989.

Since 1985, **Dr. Caroline Leaf**, a communication pathologist and audiologist, has worked in the area of cognitive neuroscience. She has specialized in traumatic brain injury (TBI) and learning disabilities, focusing specifically on the science of thought as it pertains to thinking and learning. She developed The Geodesic Information Processing Theory and did some of the initial research in neuroplasticity back in the 1990s, showing how the mind can change the brain. A large part of her research in recent years has been to link scientific principles with Scripture, showing how science is catching up with the Bible.

She applied the findings of her research in clinical practice for nearly twenty years and now lectures and preaches around the world on these topics. She is a prolific author of many books, articles, and scientific articles. She has been a featured guest of *Enjoying Everyday Life* with Joyce Meyer; *LIFE Today* with James and Betty Robison; Marilyn Hickey; Sid Roth; and TBN's *Doctor to Doctor*, among many others. She now hosts her own show on TBN called *Switch On Your Brain*.

Leaf's passion is to help people see the link between science and Scripture as a tangible way of controlling their thoughts and emotions, so they can learn how to think, learn, and find their sense of purpose in life.

Caroline and her husband, Mac, live in Dallas, Texas, with their four children.

For more information, visit her website at www.drleaf.com.